nurture

nurture

A Modern Guide to Pregnancy, Birth, Early Motherhood—*and* Trusting Yourself and Your Body

ERICA CHIDI
Birth + Postpartum Doula

Illustrations by Jillian Ditner

CHRONICLE BOOKS
SAN FRANCISCO

Library of Congress Cataloging-in-Publication Data

Names: Cohen, Erica Chidi, author.
Title: Nurture : a modern guide to pregnancy, birth, early motherhood—and trusting
  yourself and your body / Erica Chidi Cohen, Doula, Ceo + Co-Founder of Loom ;
  illustrations by Jillian Ditner.
Description: San Francisco : Chronicle Books, [2017] | Includes
  bibliographical references and index.
Identifiers: LCCN 2016048766 | ISBN 9781452152639 (pb : alk. paper)
Subjects: LCSH: Pregnancy—Popular works. | Childbirth—Popular works. |
  Motherhood—Popular works.
Classification: LCC RG551 .C64 2017 | DDC 618.2—dc23 LC record available at
  https://lccn.loc.gov/2016048766

Manufactured in China

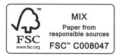

Designed by Jennifer Tolo Pierce.
Illustrations by Jillian Ditner.

10 9 8 7

Chronicle Books LLC
680 Second Street
San Francisco, California 94107
www.chroniclebooks.com

*To the mothers who have welcomed me
on their profound journey, you will forever be
my greatest teachers.*

Contents

———

Introduction

———

While writing this book, I thought a lot about you and what you might want out of a book about pregnancy, birth, and early motherhood. I considered the excitement, nervousness, exuberance, fear—a mix of potent emotions that can make you feel knocked out one minute and utterly elated the next—pregnancy brings with it. I wanted this book to help bolster you through that emotional roller coaster, providing a modern and customizable and, most importantly, judgment-free approach to this new stage of your life.

Whether you're currently pregnant or hoping to become pregnant, the constant negotiation of new feelings and experiences can be overwhelming, as can the flood of information and anecdotes coming from friends, family, and even strangers.

Rest assured, you are far from alone in these feelings. Many women feel this way in the same circumstances—and now you've got me by your side to help you. As a professional doula—which comes from the Greek term for "women's helper"—I've spent the last decade helping scores of moms-to-be through pregnancy, childbirth, and early motherhood, offering physical and emotional support, friendship, and answers to their many, many questions. I help women feel more connected to their pregnancy, and to the idea and reality of becoming a mother. In doing so, I consider the whole woman—not just her medical record. I consider how she sees herself in the world, how she takes care of herself (including rest, diet, sleep, and emotional nourishment), and what's happening to her body and the baby growing within. I provide her with unconditional support and help her translate the influx of information barreling toward her at every turn. I also encourage her to turn inward, away from the noise, and tune in to herself, to trust her intuition and focus less on the small stuff—such as the color of the nursery or which bottles to use—and focus more on being in the present moment. I introduce her to the powerful physical and emotional boosts that food can offer, and I guide her through recipes to nourish her mind, her body, and her growing baby. I also educate her on her many birthing options, and then gently help her plot out the most supportive path to her baby's arrival—while also giving her tools to use if things don't go as she anticipated.

And throughout this book, I share with you the same information, tips, and techniques that I offer clients through my doula practice. I will help you confidently navigate the coming year, while bringing you the comfort and inspiration necessary not just to forge through but also to embrace this unique time in your life.

So, why should you invite me along on your journey to motherhood? I am a caregiver by nature, and I was born into a family of caregivers. My father is a doctor, my mother is a nurse, and my paternal grandmother, someone I've always felt a connection with, was a midwife. When I was growing up, my father often told me I had an uncanny likeness to his mother, from our personality traits to our appearance. Although we never met (she passed away long before I was born), I like to think I grew up drawing from her nurturing qualities. When I was a little girl, my parents called me "Nne," which means "mother" or "grandmother" in their native Nigerian language of Igbo. My parents trained me early on in the art of caring for others, and I was driven to pursue caregiving as my own profession. Early in my career, after exploring a few different fields including the culinary arts, I moved to San Francisco, where I started volunteering at a women's health clinic. At first I was an intake assistant, welcoming women of all ages, answering their health-related questions, and connecting them with the best provider for their needs. Spanning topics from periods to menopause, I quickly gained a broad knowledge of the women's health world, including midwifery, the profession that serves a woman through pregnancy, birth, and the weeks and months following the birth. When I came upon the term "doula" and learned about the doula's role, I instantly felt my calling. It seemed to me that doulas were the missing link in the birthing experience—an adjunct to the medical model that could fill in the gaps by educating and guiding new mothers through all aspects of their transition to motherhood. Inspired by the impact I could have on others, I made the commitment to become a doula myself.

After I completed my doula training, I began my work as a solo practitioner in San Francisco, focusing on birth and postpartum client care, and incorporating my love for cooking by providing trimester-appropriate meal preparation for my clients in their homes. Clients were drawn to my unique holistic approach, and I quickly found myself with a busy practice. Years later, I moved with my husband to Los Angeles, where I started holding monthly educational workshops in our bungalow and serving nurturing meals for expectant and new mothers. These gatherings, which grew and grew, became the genesis of LOOM, a company creating education, services, and community for expecting and new parents. I cofounded it with the intention of offering a more dynamic and holistic approach to the experience.

This book is an extension of my practice. I offer it to you to help make your experience of pregnancy and motherhood feel entirely connected to the rest of your life instead of feeling like a departure from everything you have come to know. Reading these pages, you will discover simple ways to nurture yourself as you and your baby grow through the months, along with how to approach the first few weeks postpartum. You'll also learn what to expect at every stage of your pregnancy, and a flexible and blended approach to birthing options, labor, breastfeeding and nourishing your baby, plus baby care. I'll share nourishing foods and recipes for each trimester and the postpartum shift, and self-care strategies—including mindfulness techniques and self-reflection exercises—to help boost your intuition, reduce stress, and cultivate balance throughout your pregnancy and into early motherhood. I hope to teach you how to support yourself, to empower yourself to make informed decisions that spring directly out of your own personal beliefs, and to ask yourself a few tough questions. For this reason, I've intentionally designed this as a hands-on workbook. Try to interact with this book as much as you can—make it a tool in your toolbox, helping you work through the challenges and victories you'll experience on your journey. I've always found this process is best when it's a conversation, not a lecture. The moment you become a mother is one of the most significant events of your life. With this book as your guide, you'll be present for every moment, in both mind and body, not swept up by fear. You'll discover there is no "right" way to be pregnant, give birth, or mother—there's only your way. You'll learn to trust and be gentle with yourself. You'll come to know what I know to be true: You've got this.

PART ONE

Welcoming Change

In the coming chapters, we'll be looking at the incredible journey you will take to becoming a mother. We're going to save all the facts, figures, and diagrams for later, and for now, keep the focus on you. What does this pregnancy and path to motherhood mean to you, mean for you? We'll dig in and reflect on some things that, frankly, most women don't spend enough time on. We're also going to exercise a few of your self-care muscles that will help support you through your pregnancy, your labor, and maybe the rest of your life.

Welcoming change, especially those changes that come with new motherhood, can be challenging. You may not even know where to begin. Begin with yourself. In the coming pages, I encourage you to explore your environment, get to know yourself better, and look at the areas of your life beyond your own body that are about to change. Once you learn the skills that I teach you and incorporate them into your life, you'll be able to wholly welcome these changes, rather than feeling that you are just adapting to them. You'll feel curious, grounded, and empowered. Let's begin.

CHAPTER ONE

You've Got This

Ready or not, change is on its way. Throughout this book, I will be reminding you of your own strengths, your natural ability to shoulder what's about to come. You'll learn how to truly check in and read what's going on with yourself, so that you can have the fortitude and peace of mind to carry on with pregnancy, birth, and, eventually, motherhood.

It all starts with self-knowledge. In this chapter, you will explore how to adjust your perspective, develop a new emotional language, and cope with your true, raw emotions—skills that are uncannily empowering during this unique time in your life.

TUNE IN TO YOURSELF

Yes, you've got this, but you might not hear this very often—or often enough. On the contrary, you're probably hearing a lot of questions or opinions from well-intentioned friends and family: "Are you nervous?" "Where are you going to give birth?" "You have to try hypnobirthing!" Remember, these people are excited for you, but they don't know you like you do. Set all their commentary aside and start tuning in to yourself.

Throughout your pregnancy, birthing, and parenting experience, you might be told that you don't know what's best for you or your baby. But here's the thing: You do. The truth is that at a fundamental level you are already completely prepared for pregnancy and childbirth. Just as your body instinctively knows what to do, your mind does as well. The key is to remember that there is no single "right way" to experience it; rather, every way is the right way. Your experience will be yours alone, and I encourage you to embrace how it might differ from what is perceived to be the norm. The benefits of doing so—of tapping into your intuition, building your confidence in your decision-making, and releasing yourself from the burden of other people's experiences and opinions—are immeasurable.

I often speak about the concept of intuition. We've all got it—it's that gut feeling; that visceral tug of emotion that hints at what steps or actions we should take; that voice that sometimes makes the rational, logical, or easy choice seem "off." Throughout the coming months of pregnancy—and years of motherhood—when innumerable options will be presented to you, you're going to need easy access to your intuition. To gain and maintain that access, you need to stay curious and open to whatever emotions may pop up for you. (I'll teach you how to do this in the sections ahead.) By maintaining a neutral, positive, and open-minded stance, you'll allow your own intuition to guide you and your baby. And with time and practice, you'll know the saying to be true: You've got this!

POP AND THE FEELINGS CIRCLE

No doubt you've found yourself in this situation at one time or another: You're moving through your day, living life as normal, when you're called upon to make a decision—it could be as small as, say, what to have for dinner. Instantly, you feel your body tense up as emotions begin to arise. You might dismiss the tension, not wanting to analyze it (in part because analyzing it could lead you to discover an even bigger problem that needs to be dealt with or an even bigger decision that needs to be made); or you let the tension increase by allowing your mind to wander to other things that might be causing stress in your life, which creates a spinout of emotion and causes you to lose track of what prompted the initial feeling of tension. Both of these responses are very common and completely natural; indeed, our mental processes and emotions can act as defense mechanisms, protecting us from emotions that are even more unpleasant than the ones that make us initially tense up. But just because these responses are natural doesn't mean they're always helpful to us. When we brush aside our feelings or mindlessly allow our thoughts to wander, we're missing out on a chance for valuable self-reflection. As a pregnant woman, mother, and partner, you're going to find it helpful to learn to slow down your mental processes and mindfully acknowledge tension and emotions as you feel them—before they have a chance to morph into something more harmful and confusing. This will clear a path for your intuition and enable you to make more intentional decisions. After all, how can you know the right decision for you if you can't earnestly and totally tap into what you actually feel?

The next time you find yourself in the midst of tension or emotion, give POP a try. POP is a very simple mental exercise I developed to help my clients manage their emotions. POP stands for Pause; Onboard a feeling; Proceed with awareness.

The first step is easy enough: Pause. All you have to do is simply stop what you're doing when you notice the onset of the emotion.

Second, Onboard a feeling—that is, identify the emotion and allow yourself to feel it. Don't dismiss it, don't push it away, and don't let it spiral into a mix of emotions. Acknowledge that, whatever it is, it's OK, because it's part of your natural experience. If you're having trouble identifying what the feeling is—hey, it's not easy—here's a good place to start: the Feelings Circle. Most of us have a limited emotional vocabulary—meaning we're not always able to explain exactly what we're feeling, which can heighten the intensity of our negative emotions as we become frustrated by not being able to find the words to explain them. The Feelings Circle can help us clearly identify how we are feeling at any particular moment, which is a necessary starting place for processing our emotions and reducing the intensity of our experiences—skills that will be invaluable to you throughout pregnancy and childbirth.

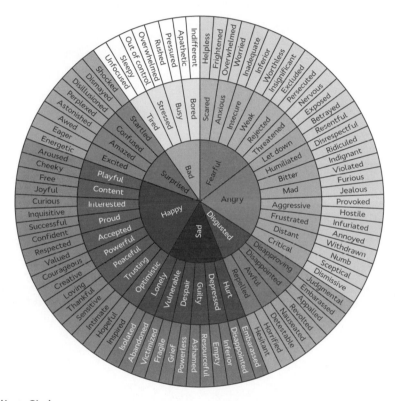

The Feelings Circle

Here's how it works: When a feeling starts to arise, look at the wheel, start with the inner-most wheel and move outward, moving from the core feelings toward any associated feelings that might be coming up for you. Alternatively, if a core emotion is not clear, you can move from the outside in, identifying the associated feeling first and then making your way toward the core emotion. Don't necessarily "hunt" for the right word. Rather, as you look, notice which words resonate with you. Another way to use the chart is to compare how you're feeling today with how you felt earlier today or even yesterday. For example: I'm feeling _____ today, but yesterday I felt _____ and _____. Typically, you might find that two or even four different emotions apply.

Having identified the emotion you're feeling, you're ready for the final step of POP: Proceed with awareness. In other words, now that you know what you truly feel, consider what action to take, or what action not to take. For example, you have a long-standing date to meet a friend for dinner. You're at the restaurant and have ordered a salad because you're hungry and she's twenty minutes late. Then you get a text from her that she has to cancel because she forgot to calendar your date and now something has come up. It's time to POP—especially before you respond to that text. You'll find that your decision will be much more intentional; this is especially helpful during pregnancy and childbirth, when emotions run high.

A Quick Vocabulary Tune-Up

Using intellectual language—words that are not connected to your direct experience—can distance you from your emotions and make it more difficult to know what you are truly feeling. To avoid this, try using simpler, more self-expressive words (emotional language) to explain what you feel. Here are some examples of emotional words you can say in place of intellectual ones:

Emotional Language	Intellectual Language
Help	Aid
Hard	Challenging
Round	Circular
Small	Diminutive
Tired	Fatigued
Hopeless	Futile
Watch	Observe
Enough	Sufficient
End	Terminate

EDITING YOUR SCRIPT

Each of us has been rehearsing a role and its lines for most of our lives. These lines are the phrases we repeat about ourselves, both positive and negative. They can reinforce truths that we hold about ourselves, but at times they are limiting. They hold us back and prevent us from being open to new possibilities about our lives and about ourselves fundamentally. They are not truths, they are not facts—they are the things we tell ourselves that keep us in "our place." Here are some examples of limiting or toxic lines in our scripts:

- I'm not creative.

- I'm not enough.

- I won't be loved if I express how I really feel.

- Something is wrong with me.

- I can't manifest what I want.

- I can't have a baby and a career.

- I'm so busy I don't have any time to slow down.

- Life is hard and always will be; I just have to get used to it.

- My mom and my grandmother had challenging labors, so I guess I will too.

- My parents are divorced, so maybe my relationship won't last.

- This pregnancy might not be easy.

Pregnancy is a prime opportunity to edit your script, because you're already moving through an incredible change. Why not change the way you talk to yourself, and the way you talk about yourself? Editing your script and moving from a negative internal conversation into a more positive one is a huge part of feeling that you've got this.

How to Edit Your Script

Look back at your history. Here I've divided your life into several stages and facets, each followed by the headings "The Good" and "The Challenging." Try reflecting on each of these sections, identifying what script you may have used at the time—and potentially a script you currently use when looking back. Feel free to write these scripts in a journal or on a piece of paper outside of this book. Don't be surprised if you find you're writing down more challenging experiences than good ones. It's important to be honest about these emotions and let them come through.

> **Birth** *(What do you know about your own birth? If possible, find out details from your mother and ask her to describe what was good and/or challenging for her. Having an understanding of your own birth and any values your mother or family might have around pregnancy or the birthing process can help you understand your journey toward giving birth. If you're unable to get this information, skip this stage.)*

The Good _____

_____

_____

The Challenging _____

_____

_____

Childhood

The Good _____

_____

_____

The Challenging _____

_____

_____

Teenage Years

The Good _____

_____

_____

The Challenging _____

_____

_____

Eighteen and Older

The Good _____

_____

_____

The Challenging _____

_____

_____

Relationships

The Good _____

_____

_____

The Challenging _____

_____

_____

Work

The Good _____

_____

_____

The Challenging _____

_____

_____

Adulthood

The Good _____

_____

_____

The Challenging _____

_____

_____

Once you are done with the exercise, acknowledge those facets of your life you identified as challenging—then leave them behind. Wish them well; they're not part of your new script. Compile all of your good experiences and transfer them into your new script on the next page.

As you let go of your challenging emotions, let this mantra guide your thoughts:

I am not my past; I am unfolding in every moment.

Your New Script

Choose at least three positive lines from your past scripts that you want to add to your new script. Then, add new lines you would like to be central to your updated script. And finally, take the most important step: Start sharing it with others.

_____

_____

_____

_____

_____

_____

_____

_____

_____

_____

_____

_____

Mama Mantra
Hug your
mistakes and celebrate
your failures.

CHAPTER TWO

Tools for Welcoming Change

———

Until you become pregnant for the first time, your body has always been only your own. Every decision you have made for your body has been motivated by your own needs and desires (possibly as influenced by societal expectations, media images, and peer pressure—still, the only person directly affected by your decisions was you). When you learn that you're pregnant, suddenly you are motivated in two different (and sometimes opposing) directions as you begin to consider, "What's best for me and what's best for my baby?" It can take time to find balance in your mind—which may be the only part that still feels like you—and your body, which begins devoting more and more of itself to the needs of your baby.

This change and this duality can be overwhelming to reconcile at first. You might be thinking, "I know I'm pregnant, but I don't feel like I know what I'm doing yet." Feeling directionless and adrift is normal. In fact, that's exactly how you're supposed to feel. Being pregnant is an opportunity for self-renewal. It's about discovering a new way to be in your body and in the world around you, while also literally being the home for your growing baby.

In the following sections, you'll find tools to help you navigate the changes ahead. I've addressed changes and challenges that are likely to arise in all sectors of your life—changes that are common for pregnant women (especially with a first pregnancy) and new mothers. As this new phase of your life unfolds, you may even want to revisit some of the ideas mentioned here. As with any transition, this one will be smooth in some places and not so smooth in others. As always, be gentle, stay curious, and try to be patient with the process. You'll start feeling like yourself—whomever that ends up being—very soon.

TOOLS FOR YOUR MIND

I've discussed the idea that before you became pregnant, you may not have pushed for exactly what you needed. You may not have felt the need to question your point of view or look deeper into yourself, either. With pregnancy, much of that can change. You may find yourself either full of self-doubt or imbued with a sense of bottomless confidence. To help you get into a healthy pregnancy mind-set, here are some simple mental tips and exercises you can do.

Release judgment and be gentle on yourself. As you and your baby grow, you might find yourself too tired to tackle simple things on your to-do list, like laundry or dishes, which may have been easy for you before pregnancy. Or maybe you'll find yourself replacing your green smoothies with a less-healthy option like grilled cheese sandwiches. It's OK. Create space for imperfection; in fact, welcome it. Becoming a mother is in part about releasing the need for control and accepting yourself just as you are.

Begin connecting with your baby. Growing babies need love and connection—these are vital nutrients. An easy way to develop a connection with your baby is to place your hands on your belly and take three deep breaths while imagining that your baby can sense your thoughts and feel your presence in that moment. Then share something with her. Speak to her, or sing to her, or simply say your thoughts out loud. At first you might feel silly or a little self-conscious; don't let that hinder you. Do this once a day, and over time a natural intimacy will begin to develop between you and your baby. Soon you might find yourself doing this multiple times a day. And when you do, listen closely, for you might feel your baby share something with you.

Ask questions. As you move through your pregnancy, you will have many questions—about your pregnant body, your baby, your relationship with your partner, nutrition, and more. Seek out a trustworthy and intelligent source to share your questions with. This could be your doctor, midwife, or doula. It could also be a friend who has already been through the process of pregnancy and childbirth. Asking questions can release stress, even if you don't get the exact answer you're looking for.

Trust yourself. Support from family and friends is important, and your community will want to help you through your journey. But don't forget to tune in to yourself and trust your intuition. You know what's best for your body and your baby. Nourish your inner trust, and you will find yourself mothering your baby in a way that feels aligned with your true self.

Flex your "no muscle." Get comfortable with saying no, not because you're selfish, but because saying it is a fundamental part of self-care. As women, many of us grew up hearing that we need to "be polite," which for some can evolve into an inability to say no or feeling valued only if we are compliant and helpful. Never saying no—or not saying it often enough—makes you exhausted, dissatisfied, and irritable. It also leaves zero room for spontaneity and space to recharge, both of which you need during your pregnancy and early motherhood. Strengthening your no muscle helps you create better boundaries for yourself and lets you make space for more of what you need. Starting off isn't easy, but here are few ways to begin integrating a little more no into your life.

- **Get clear:** Clarify what's most important to you. Discern how and where and with whom you prefer to spend most of your time. Knowing what you love and want more of will help you say no with confidence. This is the first step to master.

- **Start training:** Choose some simple, low-impact environments and situations in which to practice saying no. Maybe in an exercise class, say no to a certain movement if you feel your body isn't up for it, instead of pushing yourself. Say no when someone tries to sell you something on the street or you get offered a sample at the grocery store. Or go into a room by yourself, shut the door, and say no out loud ten times. It sounds slightly silly, but it can help.

- **FOMO:** For some of us, the hardest part of saying no will be Fear of Missing Out. Sure, saying no leads to a missed opportunity. But reframe it; think of it as a trade-off. Remind yourself that when you're saying no, you are potentially saying yes to something better, even if you don't know what it is yet. Deny the ask, not the person: When you do say no, thank them for thinking of you or asking for your involvement. You're not rejecting the person. Make that clear. Let them know that you respect or admire them and the work they are doing, or the event or activity you're being invited to. Let them know that the *no* is not personal. For example: "This sounds amazing but my plate is so full. Have a great time, and circle back again the next time something like this comes up."

- **Be brave:** If you're someone who is used to saying yes, saying no will feel bad at first. You may feel like a terrible friend or family member. You might feel like you're letting someone down or not living up to expectations, or that people will see you in a negative light. Try and push through these initial feelings; with time and a little bravery, they will recede and be replaced by the happiness found in doing more of the things you love.

TOOLS FOR YOUR BODY

Throughout pregnancy, it may well be assumed—by your doctor or midwife, many books, even a birth class—that you have a fairly solid understanding of female anatomy. After working with many, many new mothers, I can level with you here: Some of us forgot this stuff the day our high school biology exam ended (if we even knew it then!), and we haven't looked back. Once you're pregnant, if you feel there are important gaps in your knowledge, you'll need to get up to speed again; knowing how your body works is integral to knowing how best to support it. What's more, once you know the amazing intricacies of your reproductive system, you may even feel empowered by it. So let's review.

Vagina Although the vagina is commonly thought of as an open tunnel, it's actually the opposite—it's a collapsed muscular tube. The walls touch; it's a flexible duct providing an easy pathway for your period, sexual intercourse, and the delivery of your baby.

Uterus Many people don't know that the uterus is actually a muscle—and an incredibly strong one at that. It's made up of multiple muscle layers that are capable of expanding or stretching to accommodate your baby and releasing your baby into the world through contractions during labor. It's situated between your bladder and your rectum, shaped like an inverted pear and about the size of a small fist (prebaby). The uterus is made up of three segments: the fundus, which is the upper portion; the body, which is the large central portion; and the cervix, the narrow lower portion shaped like the end of a balloon.

Cervix Although the cervix is technically part of the uterus, it works so hard during pregnancy that it deserves its own description. It remains tightly closed throughout pregnancy to hold in your baby, amniotic fluid, and all the other uterine contents. During labor, it dilates (opens) and effaces (thins), to allow your baby to make his way through the birth canal.

Urethra This tube runs from your bladder to just in front of the vaginal opening (vulva) and allows for the passage of urine. Although it's not a sexual or reproductive organ, it's located very close to your vagina and uterus, which means that it can be affected by pregnancy. For example, as your baby grows, this can place extra pressure on the bladder and the urethra, so you need to go to the bathroom more frequently or have less control over the urge to pee.

Ovaries and fallopian tubes Your fallopian tubes extend from either side of your uterus, each arching over an ovary. Your ovaries contain all of your eggs from the time that you were six months in utero. Each month, ovulation releases an egg (or eggs) from the ovary; it enters the fallopian tube, where it may be fertilized. (Rarely, a fertilized ovum implants in the fallopian tube, causing an ectopic pregnancy and requiring emergency treatment.) The egg continues to the uterus, where if fertilized it will implant and grow; if not fertilized, it is eliminated along with that month's uterine lining as menstrual flow.

Pelvis The pelvis is a flexible cradle that provides a foundation for your pelvic muscles and contains your pelvic organs. Your pelvis has two corresponding halves, each with three prominent bones—the ischium, the ileum, and the pubis (pubic bone). They are connected by ligaments to the sacrum coccyx, the bones that form the lower end of your spine. In pregnancy these joints become even more mobile, allowing your pelvis to open and make space for your growing baby.

Pelvic floor The muscles of the pelvis are arranged much like the strands of a woven basket, forming a strong carriage called the pelvic floor. These muscles stretch from the bottom edge of your pubic bone to the back of your sacrum. Along the sides they attach to the inner and bottom edges of the pelvis. Your urethra passes through the pelvic floor, as do the vagina and the rectum. The front group of pelvic floor muscles helps prevent unintentional urination; the rear group helps prevent unintentional bowel movements. These muscles support the vagina and other structures within the pelvis that are controlled both voluntarily and involuntarily.

Perineum The perineum is a smooth, roughly diamond-shaped area of skin between the vaginal opening and the anus, connected to the muscles of the pelvic floor on all sides. It's both tough and pliant, allowing it to stretch and adapt to the needs of childbirth.

Breasts The breasts are modified sweat glands with the amazing potential to produce milk. Each breast comprises mostly fatty tissue, with twelve to twenty-five lobes radiating around the nipple. Each lobe contains clusters of alveoli, the glands that produce and store milk. Ducts surround the lobes and are covered by smooth muscles that contract to allow milk to be ejected from your nipple, in the center of the darker pigmented area called the areola. The skin that surrounds your nipple might be a little bumpy. These bump-like protrusions, called Montgomery tubercles, lubricate the areola and maintain an acidic pH, which helps prevent bacterial growth if you choose to breastfeed.

TOOLS FOR THE TOUGHER STUFF

A wanted pregnancy is most certainly a joyful thing. And yet, for a mother, it can also be a time of complicated emotions. I will venture to say that all women who experience pregnancy will, at some point, have to confront strong feelings about this enormous change—to their body, to their lifestyle, to their everyday dealings. And many women—maybe even you—may also have to confront painful issues from their past that can be easily triggered during pregnancy.

You may have already taken the time and decided to acknowledge these traumas through therapy, support groups, or within your community, or maybe this is the first time you felt it was necessary to move through and beyond the pain. Wherever you may fall on this spectrum, if something is coming up for you, I urge you to take stock of your support systems and get what you need from them. Pregnancy, and eventually your relationship with your baby, can be healing.

Pregnancy Loss

This may not be your first pregnancy. Perhaps you've experienced a miscarriage, a stillbirth, or an abortion. In fact, 8 to 20 percent of women who know they are pregnant have a miscarriage some time before twenty weeks of pregnancy; 80 percent of these occur in the first twelve weeks (http://www.uptodate.com/contents/miscarriage-beyond-the-basics). If this is the case, you may find yourself dealing with challenging emotions at various stages of this pregnancy. You may pass a time marker that was a turning point in the past, when a certain test came in or the week you lost your baby, for example. Even with a healthy baby born to term, some women still feel grief for their lost baby postpartum. These times will undoubtedly be difficult. You might not want to talk about your pregnancy when you first confirm it; you may decide to share your good news much later, if at all. All of these feelings are normal. I would still encourage you to address them and talk with your partner, counselor, coach, doula, or therapist. Grief is a process that runs on a continuum. There is no right amount of time, antidote, or correct way to do it. Connecting with someone you trust can help lighten the journey.

Start talking. This may be the last thing you want to do, and I completely understand that. If you do choose to share your experience, more often than not you will discover similar stories within your own community—friends, colleagues, or family members may come forward to share their story. Don't underestimate the healing power of connecting with your community.

Find a group. If you're not ready to talk to your community and you'd like to keep some anonymity, group therapy is a great option. Many different associations offer meetings (some have church or community affiliations, if that helps). Visit nationalshare.org for a list of support resources, including Facebook groups.

Go online. There are online groups in the form of storytelling resources and message boards. This may be just the thing you need for immediate and round-the-clock support. If you're seeking pregnancy loss support and education, throughtheheart.org is a good place to start.

Get into your body. Acupuncture or bodywork like Mayan abdominal massage, or even energy work like Reiki and craniosacral therapy, can help you process the physical and emotional grief in your body and complement any talk or group therapy you are doing.

Sexual Abuse

One in five women will experience some form of sexual abuse at some point in her life, whether in childhood or adulthood (www.nsvrc.org/sites/default/files/publications_nsvrc_factsheet_media-packet_statistics-about-sexual-violence_0.pdf). While sexual trauma is alarmingly common, the aftereffects can vary greatly from person to person. Typically, they last a long time, and many of the dynamics of pregnancy, labor, and delivery can act as triggers. A vaginal exam or other vaginal procedure is one of the most common triggers; birth pain, especially in the vagina, but also in the abdomen, perineum, low back, and breasts, can also be triggering. A patient's relationship to her care provider, who can be seen as an authority figure, may remind a survivor of her perpetrator; this can make her feel powerless or submissive. In labor and birth, and in the cultural space around it, you'll hear a lot of discussion about "giving in" to contractions and pain. That idea can also be triggering for survivors, who may associate retaining control with their safety. Memories or flashbacks can come rushing in at these times; however, some women's trauma manifests itself unconsciously in the form of anger, tension, or illness. If you have suffered abuse, you will want to be aware of both of these potential results.

As in the case of pregnancy loss, I encourage you to talk about your feelings as they appear (look to POP and the Feelings Circle, page 15, for a refresher on tuning in to your feelings). You may want to take stock ahead of time—line up a friend, therapist, or other trusted person you can call on if you need them.

Allow your feelings to exist. Know that they are normal; that they make sense; that they are valid. Very rarely does sexual abuse leave survivors free from aftereffects, so know that you are right and that these feelings are to be expected.

Consider working with a therapist who specializes in navigating trauma. Many will have experience with motherhood and survivors—be sure to ask about this in a preliminary meeting.

If authority is triggering for you, look for a care provider you are comfortable talking to about your trauma. You don't have to be specific if you don't want to be. Many care providers in the birth space are familiar with the needs of survivors and can support you through your pregnancy.

I encourage you to work with a doula you trust, one who is also familiar with the needs of survivors. Again, you don't have to be specific about your abuse if you don't want to be—just let your doula know about your fears and concerns so she can help you navigate them and provide emotional support.

If you have a partner or other trusted support person, look to them during this time. Be specific about what tests or exams make you uncomfortable, and work with them in advance.

Domestic Violence and Abuse

Abuse can take many forms—physical, emotional, verbal, psychological, and others—and it can create a confusing, stressful, and painful environment for its sufferers. That is the goal of the abuser, in addition to making you feel ashamed, powerless, hopeless, or isolated. When you're pregnant, abuse can bring additional risks, such as high blood pressure, vaginal bleeding, nausea and vomiting, premature birth, or a baby who may need intense medical support after birth. Domestic violence also puts you at higher risk of death during pregnancy. If you are suffering from abuse, know this: It is not your fault. Leaving an abusive partner can be extremely difficult, especially with your baby as an added concern. You deserve a positive pregnancy, birth, and motherhood. Whether or not you do decide to make a change, there are many resources available to support you.

Turn to someone you trust. A great first step can be turning to a friend, family member, or colleague whom you trust. Especially if you're feeling hopeless, an ally can help you sort out what your next steps could be.

Turn to a professional. If you're comfortable opening up to your OB, midwife, doula, or counselor, they could be helpful in determining how best to help you.

Contact a national agency. The phone number for the National Domestic Violence Hotline is easy to remember for a reason—commit it to memory and call when you need someone to talk to or you'd like to discuss local resources, including an escape plan. The number is 1-800-799-HELP (7233).

TOOLS FOR YOUR RELATIONSHIPS

During your pregnancy and as you welcome your baby into your life, her presence will naturally shift your other relationships. All of a sudden this new being has appeared and, as if out of nowhere, become the axis around which everything else spins. Aside from your partner, this little baby is now your number one relationship—and that can be quite a change for both you and your community. Navigating that shift can be tough and even painful as your focus shifts and changes from what you've previously known. It can be hard to find the confidence to leave behind the way things once were, but a certain amount of fluidity and communication can really help.

Your Partner

Partner relationships are tricky on their own—we've all dealt with a certain degree of drama, I am sure. Add pregnancy and a new baby into the mix, even with a solid relationship, and things can escalate. Numerous studies indicate that, on average, couples' satisfaction decreases after the birth of their first child and continues to decrease with each additional child. That doesn't have to be you, though, especially if you actively decide to prioritize your relationship. In fact, a growing number of hospitals, midwives, and doulas are teaching relationship skills alongside childbirth education classes. Just think: The best way to model a good, respectful relationship for your baby is to have one yourself. Here are a few ways to ease the transition and establish a firm foundation during pregnancy.

First person first. Share how you're feeling with your partner using "I" statements, which tend to make the speaker take responsibility for their emotions. This makes sense; after all, we can truly know only our own feelings. When we talk about anyone else's feelings, thoughts, or behaviors ("you don't love me" or "you don't understand"), we're just assuming these things are true. Share what you know—yourself—and wait openly for your partner's answer.

Read together. Find books or articles on parenting that you can read together and discuss. You could even both download a pregnancy app that details each week's progress, then read about your growing baby together. Activities like these are the basis of great coparenting and draw you closer together as you truly feel that creating this baby is something you're doing together.

Go to your appointments together. Ask your partner to attend as many appointments as he or she can. This can help your partner feel more plugged in with you and your baby's progress, and better learn how to support you along the way. (Remember to use "I" language when describing why your partner's presence is important to you.)

Take stock. Review your relationship duties and assumptions ahead of time. So often, relationship conflicts arise around dividing up and keeping score of who does what. This is intensified by the presence of a new baby who needs so much more from you both. Make a detailed list of the mundane things—bills, diapers, garbage—and the not so mundane—how religious beliefs and practices, ethics, and values will figure into your child-rearing, how to make time for each other—and figure out exactly how you plan to make things work. (A note: Even if you don't execute all of this as planned, this is a great exercise!)

Some Starter Questions for Taking Stock

- What does parenting mean to each of us?

- What did we love about how we were parented?

- How are we financially supporting ourselves and our child?

- How are we going to split parenting duties? What duties excite you? Get specific.

- What kind of postpartum support or childcare do we need?

- How important is religion and spirituality to us, in terms of our pregnancy, and how will we bring it into our parenting?

- How will we make time for each other, our passions, and our self-care (sex, date nights, and so on)?

Talk to someone—together. A study published in 2006 in the *Journal of Consulting and Clinical Psychology* showed that expectant couples and new parents who participated in weekly group counseling or coaching meetings experienced a much smaller decline in relationship satisfaction over five years compared with parents who didn't have the counseling or coaching. Counseling isn't only for marriages on the rocks—if you're open to it, it can help you become or stay aligned.

A note about sex. Pregnancy increases the blood flow to your pelvic area, which can increase sexual pleasure or make you more sensitive than usual. Make sure you are communicating to your partner what you are feeling.

If you're single . . . I encourage you to look into your community to find a partner—no, not romantically. A best friend, a sister, a colleague, even your mother could be the support you need during pregnancy and birth. She can come with you to appointments, help build nursery furniture, and even attend your birth, if you want.

Your Friends

Depending on the stage of your life that you find yourself in, pregnancy will have widely differing effects on your friendships. Maybe you're the last of your close friends to become pregnant, and you feel like you're finally one of the group again; maybe everyone is pregnant at the same time, and your friends are the allies and support they've always been; or maybe you're the first of your circle to become pregnant and you feel isolated and different. Maybe your situation is like none of these. Whatever your experience, there is likely to be some element of change as you lose extra time and mental bandwidth to devote to your friendships. Here are several proactive ways to negotiate these transitions.

Choose your own adventure. You may find yourself out with your friends as they enjoy cocktails—and feeling that this is less fun for you than it used to be. Or at a party, searching for the nearest chair. That's natural—you shouldn't expect yourself to keep up your former interest or stamina while pregnant. Instead of trying to go with the flow, why not suggest some activities or plans that interest you more? Invite that friend who's a fabulous cook to a knife skills or cooking class; look into drawing classes with another friend; plan movie nights, a book club, whatever interests you. Start with the activity and then recruit your friends.

Turn them into aunties and uncles. Take a page from corporate America: People love title changes. Seriously, though, if you involve your friends in your new transition, they might surprise you. Maybe you'll get an encouraging text before an exam you've been stressed about, or they'll be the ones to bring you magazines if you're on bed rest. Give it a shot; actively involving your friends in your pregnancy and new motherhood may add new depth to your friendship.

Be understanding, flexible, and patient. If you're feeling isolated, know that it's normal and that you won't feel this way forever. Fear of Missing Out (FOMO) can be at an all-time high during this time, as Instagram, Snapchat, Facebook—sheesh, even Periscope—let us know where our friends are and all the fun they're undoubtedly having. You can't change how they'll act, but you can change your point of view. Try to be understanding—they can't be expected to change their lives simply because you are changing yours! Be flexible—adapt where you can, retreat where you can't. And finally, be patient—it can take friends time to come to terms with your shifting priorities.

Ask how they feel. This can feel like foreign territory, given how much pregnancy is about the mother, but checking in with your friends to ask them how they feel about the upcoming transition can be very therapeutic. See it from their side, and be the support you seek.

Build your mother community. If you don't already have one, definitely begin to build your community of like-minded mothers. Prenatal yoga is a great way to start meeting people; birth education classes are also helpful. If you're comfortable doing so, ask your network to introduce you to someone new. Hey, blind dates actually work!

Advice Overwhelm

You may find that being pregnant puts you on the receiving end of a lot of advice and perhaps a bit of criticism, too. You'll get some from strangers, but the comments from people you actually know tend to be the ones that echo in your mind. Sometimes the advice is helpful, but most of the time it's not. Sometimes it can really hurt. The important thing is to tap into your intuition and decide what is right for you. Try this rejoinder (either spoken or just repeated internally, while graciously nodding your head): "Good for you, just not for me or where I'm at." I'd also suggest that you pick two friends, besides your care provider and birth team, whom you want to consult for advice; then consider tuning out everyone else. Also, avoid Dr. Google; if you have burning questions, instead try consulting a living, breathing person with expertise or experience.

Your Family

Some people have television families that are all thoughtfulness, support, and frozen homemade casseroles. Most of us don't. That said, pregnancy can bring forward some strong emotions about your family, especially as you start to envision beginning your own. You could feel the urge to repair or strengthen bonds with some of them; you may reach a breaking point with others and decide it's time to take a temporary—or even a permanent—break from them. As we discussed in the introduction to this chapter, pregnancy can bring things into sharper focus for you as you decide what's best for both you and your baby. Here are some tips for navigating these relationships.

Take stock—again. Consider your close familial relationships, those who are your core—whether that's parents, steps, and siblings, or aunts, uncles, and cousins. Try to reflect on which relationships serve you and feel like they nourish and nurture you in the way that you would like. Then move on to the more difficult ones. What is valuable for you about that person? Anything? Take what you need; give what you want.

Give and take, continued. Recognize that some relationships have relied on you. Maybe you fell into a pattern of parenting a parent, for instance. With a newborn on the way, you really won't be able to fill that role anymore, and you shouldn't. If you feel comfortable, try discussing this with the family member in question. If you don't, take note mentally and begin to pare down how accessible or hands-on you are.

It's about you. Say what you need (trying to be empathetic to others' feelings), but don't expect much. People are who they are; oftentimes, repairing a relationship means learning to accept what you can and move on from what you can't.

No one gets an all-access pass. Although birth is an exciting and hotly anticipated moment for a family, no one gets backstage unless you say so. This can be tough; you may have to tell your own mother or the guardian who raised you from diapers that you don't want to share this moment with them. That's fine—you call the shots. If they don't understand or respect that, feel free to use your care provider and their protocols as a buffer, as these can be harder to disagree with. (For more on how to deal with parents and boundaries postpartum, see Your Environment, page 312.)

TOOLS FOR THE WORKPLACE

Negotiating a fruitful work-life balance isn't easy, and yours will likely morph and shift through the years. It is possible, however. You just need to be clear about what you want and need, taking into account that no one (not men, not women) can ever truly have it all. You will make choices; you will set priorities; you will set boundaries. You may not know the answer quite yet— some women realize they couldn't possibly go back to work after giving birth; others can't wait—but eventually you will. Plus, with technology as our ally, we've got more resources than ever to custom-build a supportive work environment and hopefully create a more cushioned transition.

Maternity Leave

In the United States, a patchwork of federal and state laws provides basic protections to pregnant women and their babies. Based on those laws, every working mother must piece together her own maternity leave using a combination of Short Term Disability (STD), sick days, vacation days, personal days, and, if applicable, her company's maternity days. Sadly, many American working mothers don't receive a paid maternity leave. In order to make the most of your leave, it's important that you know your rights and options. Here is a basic rundown of what resources are available and some things to consider.

FMLA Under the Family Medical Leave Act (FMLA), if you work for a company with more than fifty employees within seventy-five miles of your workplace and you meet some work requirements, you are entitled to twelve weeks of unpaid maternity leave from your company without the risk of losing your job. Assuming you have employer-sponsored health insurance, your company will also be required to pay (or partially pay) for your health insurance while you are on leave. That said, many women have to return to work before the twelve weeks, as they aren't being paid. Additionally, if you are among the top 10 percent of wage earners at your company, and your employer can prove that your absence would cause the company significant financial harm, they are not required to hold your job for your return. Thus your job may be jeopardized by your taking maternity leave (www.whattoexpect.com/pregnancy/maternity-leave).

STD Short Term Disability (STD) is financial support for your maternity leave from either your employer, union, or state. STD will typically cover your salary or a portion of it for, on average, six weeks. There is also private disability insurance you can pay into. Check the Department of Labor (dol.gov) to see what parameters apply in your state.

Give notice Federal guidelines require you to give thirty days' notice before taking your maternity leave; giving notice shortly after your first trimester is more common (and more courteous).

Human Resources Speak to your human resources department after you've completed your first trimester to discuss what options you have and what your company can offer you. For example, in some instances your company will "advance" you vacation days you have yet to accrue. Be forewarned, however, that if you choose not to return to work, you may have to reimburse the cost of those days to your company.

Speak to your boss first Tell your boss before you confide in other coworkers so she doesn't hear it through other sources. Communicate that you are dedicated to your position and plan to work until your due date, barring unforeseen circumstances.

Paternity leave Some states also offer paternity leave (also called family leave) for fathers and partners. Again, look at the Department of Labor's website to get an idea of the resources available from your state.

Insurance Assurance

Pregnancy is when many women finally get "back on the grid" and become insured. Even if you are already insured, it's a good idea to look at your coverage and compare other options. Having a baby is expensive, no matter where or how you do it, and you'll want to ensure that you have the best coverage possible within your budget. Here's a brief breakdown of the different types of health insurance available in the United States.

- **Through your employer.** The most common type of insurance is group coverage through your employer.

- **Through your spouse's employer.** If you have other insurance available through your spouse's employer, it's a good idea to compare this coverage to your own.

- **Individual or state exchange.** If you are self-employed, unemployed, or underinsured by your employer, you can purchase insurance as an individual from a private insurance company.

- **Medicaid or the Children's Health Insurance Program.** These are two great options for low-income families. Visit healthcare.gov to see if you qualify to enroll.

>>>

If the insurance system and its subtleties make your head spin, you're not alone. Here are several important questions to consider when researching insurance and deciding what coverage will be best for you and your baby.

- Does it cover both pregnancy and birth?

- Are only obstetricians covered? What about midwives? What about doulas?

- Are only hospitals covered? What about birth centers? What about home births?

- What happens in the event of a transfer from birth center to hospital?

- How much is the copayment per visit? And for your stay at the hospital or birth center?

- Does it cover prescription medication?

- Does it cover the various tests throughout pregnancy?

- What newborn care is covered?

- Are both well-child and sick visits to the pediatrician covered?

- Are required medications for your baby covered?

Returning to Work

It can be tough to leave your little baby behind when you decide to go back to work, no matter how much you love what you do. New motherhood can bring forward many new feelings; the transition can be tough, and you may be full of self-doubt, wondering if you made the best choice. Give it time and do your best to reacclimate. As with homesickness, you may find that once you get into a rhythm, these feelings fade away. If they don't, the great thing about your baby is that he's here to stay—and will be waiting at home for you. Here are some tips to navigate returning to work.

Give notice. Before you leave work, ask your boss or HR support how much notice they'll need for you to come back and if there are any procedures in place related to your reentry.

Arrange childcare. Before you return to work, line up childcare that you trust. If you're able to hire a nanny, you can source one from your community (Facebook is good for this, especially for finding local mom groups) or you can look into nanny agencies. If you already know you'll be returning to work, consider looking at daycare providers before your baby is born so that you can visit and vet several options.

Connect with your caregiver. Set up a play date (or several) with your nanny or daycare before you return to work. At twelve weeks old, your baby probably won't have much stranger anxiety yet, but you will be reassured to see them together.

Establish baby time. Once you're back at work, adjust your baby's schedule so that you see him for several hours daily. If you know you'll have to work late, get up early with your baby. Start a morning ritual of walking to the park or to get your morning coffee. Or if you're able to leave when the clock strikes five, be the one to give your baby dinner and a bedtime bath. Build these rituals into your day so you get the baby time you want.

Set boundaries at work. Have a realistic talk with your supervisor about time. If your nanny has to leave by six every night and you have to commute home, let them know you'll have to leave on time, every time. This can be tough, depending on your company's culture, so a frank discussion ahead of time is valuable.

Arrange a space for pumping. If you plan to breastfeed and you don't have a private office, discuss a good, private place for you to periodically pump. It shouldn't have to be a bathroom stall—assert to your employer that you need their real support to reach your breastfeeding goals, and make sure to check with your local legislation about workplace pumping laws and your rights. For more about continuing to breastfeed while working, check out *Work. Pump. Repeat.: The New Mom's Survival Guide to Breastfeeding and Going Back to Work* by my friend Jessica Shortall.

If You Freelance

More than one-third of the American workforce is freelance. And more than half of all freelancers in the United States are women—about 53 percent in 2015. If you're included in that demographic, you know that the freelance life is not the long brunches and hiking breaks that your office friends seem to think it is. You know that freelancing can be a 24-hour hustle cycle, with the oh-so-common fear of "never working again" looming beyond every completed project. Freelancing can seem ideal for new mothers who want control over their time and schedule—and indeed, it can be a great way to earn a living with more flexibility and autonomy—but it's not without its struggles. I would resist the urge to launch a freelance business as a new mother; give yourself six months to a year to acclimate to your baby and your new role. And for those who already freelance, let's unpack some tips on how to navigate your transition as a new working mother.

Take the time. The first and most important piece of advice I have for you is to actually plan on taking your own maternity leave (ideally, one you've saved for, so it can be a "paid" rather than an unpaid leave). You may think you'll answer emails or finish a report while your baby sleeps ('cause he'll be sleeping all the time, right?), but you'll need time to recuperate and rest as well. Plan on taking a month, at the very least.

Be up front with clients. Let regular clients know that you're pregnant and that you plan on taking a maternity leave. If you know your projects in advance, you can backlog work so that you don't miss a beat. Alternatively, well in advance you can speak to other freelancers in your field about stepping in for you during this time (with the understanding that you'll be stepping back in) and also run that idea by your clients. Having an established network of other freelancers whose work you know and trust can really pay off in this situation.

Be overly realistic. Don't load up your schedule too much or expect you'll be back in the swing of things right away. Expect to be tired, distracted, and emotional, and factor that into your planning—that way you'll find you are able to handle the lighter workload with your reduced capacity.

Pare it down and see how it goes. If your household has two incomes, try paring back your expenses ahead of time. Live as if you have only one income to rely on, and see how it goes. (You can put your earnings into a savings account for now, which will be an added bonus later.) Unless you live in California, where it's possible to pay into a state disability fund that becomes available during maternity leave, you won't have the kind of financial support you'd get from an employer's paid maternity leave or short-term disability.

App it up. Try streamlining some of your other duties so that you can get down to work when it's time. Time-saving apps like Instacart (grocery delivery), Washio (dry cleaning and laundry delivery), and TaskRabbit (help with household errands and chores) can help get things done for you.

Bring in backup. Consider hiring a nanny, enlisting the help of a family member, or working with a daycare provider to free up the time you need for your freelance work and other personal needs. That last item is important; don't feel that every moment of paid care has to be 100-percent productive (lord knows that's not the case when you're in an office). Get a regular schedule in place, whether it's every day or several days per week, and use the time as you see fit. Exercise, take a nap, see a friend.

TOOLS FOR PERSONAL AND HOME CARE

It could happen when you see your vulnerable little baby with her tender skin, or it could happen as soon as you become pregnant. Somewhere along the line, many new mothers seem to have an "aha!" moment about the chemicals that are in most of our personal and home care products. Some of these chemicals (actually, a lot of them) are banned in other countries, and many are carcinogens. According to the Environmental Working Group (EWG), the average American woman applies 168 chemicals to her body every single day. The United States government hasn't passed legislation concerning the chemicals in consumer products since 1938, and cosmetic companies aren't regulated by the FDA. Your skin is your largest organ and is a permeable barrier, which means it absorbs whatever you put on it. It just makes sense to switch to nontoxic products. For some advice on where to start and what to look for, I tapped my great friend Katey Denno, a celebrity makeup artist and green-beauty guru. Her knowledge of ingredients (both good and bad) is incredibly vast; I knew she would have strong advice for you. We're living in a time when we no longer have to sacrifice results (think shiny hair, anti-aging technology, on-trend makeup) in order to live a clean, green lifestyle. Your products don't have to be 100-percent organic (although it's nice if they are), but they should by all means be 100-percent nontoxic. Here are some of Katey's top ideas for how to "green" your cabinet.

Check Your Labels!

Ingredients	Why to Avoid Them
Parabens	Preservatives that prevent the growth of bacteria but also disrupt the normal behavior of estrogen. Linked to breast cancer. Look for methyl-, isobutyl-, propyl-, etc.
Formaldehyde	A preservative predominantly used in cosmetics and a known carcinogen. Look for quaternium-15, DMDM hydantoin, imidazolidinyl urea, diazolidinyl urea, sodium hydroxymethylglycinate, 2-bromo-2-nitropropane-1,3 diol (Bronopol).
Phthalates	Plasticizing chemicals that make products more malleable and helps fragrance stick to skin. May cause birth defects. Look for DBP, DEHP, DEP.
Diethanolamine and Triethanolamine	Known carcinogens that disrupt hormone function. Product added to soaps and cleansers to help them foam up better. Look for DEA, MEA, TEA.
Diazolidinyl Urea and Imidazolidinyl Urea	An antimicrobial preservative present in up to 20 percent of consumer products, which releases formaldehyde. Look for diazolidinyl urea or imidazolidinyl urea.

>>>

Ingredients	Why to Avoid Them
Sodium Lauryl Sulfate and Sodium Laureth Sulfate	Known skin irritants, so companies will add 1,4-dioxane, a by-product of petrochemicals (and known carcinogen) to help reduce allergic reactions. Look for SLS and SLES.
Propylene Glycol	A thickening and softening agent used in conjunction with known carcinogens 1,4-dioxane and ethylene oxide. Look for PEG.
Nanoparticles	Extremely small particles that make otherwise insoluble additives water-soluble. What does this mean? Oftentimes carcinogenic additives can be better absorbed into the skin. Nanomaterials may also be present in some foods, although this is yet to be conclusively confirmed by the FDA. Look for "(nano)" following another ingredient.
Synthetic Fragrance	Engineered fragrances can have as many as three thousand or more chemicals present, including hormone disrupters and allergens. The chemical makeup of these solutions isn't required to be disclosed, so it never is. Look for fragrance, flavor added.

Facial care This is the most-purchased category of personal care product. Just think—cleansers, toners, serums, moisturizers, masks, oils, night creams . . . there's a lot. Replacing your whole supply may feel daunting, so start by searching for your favorite products on the Environmental Working Group's cosmetic database, Skin Deep (ewg.org/skindeep), then start swapping out what you need to. Whole Foods and your local health food store are good places to start. For specific brands, check out The Goods (page 402).

Nail polish There is no reason to expose yourself to any of the highly toxic ingredients in mainstream nail polish during a mani/pedi. Try your hand at painting your own nails at home with any one of the wonderful "5-free" polishes (free of the five most harmful ingredients, including formaldehyde, that are found in mainstream polish), or bring your favorite nontoxic polish to your local nail salon. While in the salon, try sitting close to the door and ask if you can have it propped open. Limiting your time inhaling the fumes is another way to lower your overall exposure to known toxins.

Coconut oil Choose a coconut oil that's organic and unrefined, and use it for everything from body, hand, and foot moisturizer to hair conditioning treatment to eye cream. When you're pregnant, it's the perfect relief for tight skin around the belly, breasts, and thighs.

Sunscreen The best sunscreens are actually sunblocks that don't absorb into the skin. Many of the chemicals that prevent the burning or tanning that can lead to skin cancer are actually known carcinogens! Explain that logic. Look for sunblock with non-nano zinc oxide or titanium dioxide. Both are naturally broad-spectrum.

Laundry soap Most laundry detergents are made up entirely of chemicals, the worst (and most common) of which are called surfactants. These are chemical compounds that enable the detergent to better penetrate fabrics. Surfactants are known carcinogens and are also linked to reproductive disorders. And even worse, these are not rinsed out by your washing machine's rinse cycle; you'll carry them around with you all day, embedded in your clothing. Earth Friendly Products is one example of a surfactant-free brand, but you can refer to ewg.org for more recommendations.

All the rest Overhauling the products you're accustomed to using can be daunting once you realize there are harmful chemicals in almost every conventional product. That said, it's important to try, so taking it step by step is the key. Here are some other categories you should look into (check ewg.org for a detailed examination of which products you're using that could be harmful): toothpaste, lipstick/lip balm, makeup, body lotion, hair care products, soap and body wash, cleaning products, candles.

Club Med

There's a common belief that during pregnancy your body has to be free from all medications, a totally pure vessel. That's not actually true, not to mention quite the impossible standard! Do you take a prescription drug or regularly rely on an over-the-counter medicine? Many of them may be safe in pregnancy. The FDA rates all drugs to determine if they are safe to use during pregnancy. The scale starts at A (completely safe) and goes to X (as in, don't ever use anything rated X). Always discuss a new medication or a medication rated below a B with your care provider to weigh whether you should use it. If your medication is not safe to continue using during pregnancy, your care provider can also help recommend alternative options for coping.

Scat, Cat

Of all the wonderful ways in which your family, friends, and partner can support you during your pregnancy, litter box maintenance is always a favorite to delegate. You see, cat feces can contain the parasite toxoplasma gondii, which can cause toxoplasmosis, a rare but serious blood disease. Fetuses can become infected, which can lead to very serious complications, such as mental retardation, convulsions, low birth weight, brain calcification, and more. Please note: Your cat himself cannot infect you, only his solid waste, so you can keep your beloved pet around as long as you don't go near his fecal matter. Wash your hands after handling him and don't allow him up on counters or surfaces.

Mama Mantra

An unexpected challenge creates space for unexpected strength.

CHAPTER THREE

Cultivating Balance:

Easy Self-Care Practices for Every Stage of Pregnancy

———

Do you routinely practice self-care? If not, pregnancy is the perfect time to start, especially since you are not the only one who will benefit from self-care—your growing baby will, as well. Self-care is the practice of regularly setting aside time to be kind to yourself. Self-care can be as simple as taking a warm bath, calling a friend who always makes you laugh, eating a healthy snack, or going on a walk. In this chapter, I'm going to walk you through five helpful self-care practices that are especially beneficial in pregnancy: mindfulness, movement, journaling, natural remedies, and nourishment. (You'll see these practices again in Part Two, where I've woven them into the month-by-month guide for every stage of your pregnancy.) Give them a try or let them inspire you to explore your own self-care ideas; choose any activity that fuels and uplifts, and make it a regular part of your daily life.

MINDFULNESS

Mindfulness is a moment-to-moment awareness of your thoughts and the sensations you're feeling in your body. It stems from Buddhist traditions, which also promote the practice of accepting things exactly as they are without judgment. A mindfulness practice is a gentle and portable form of self-care. Studies suggest it may reduce pregnancy-related anxiety, stress, and depression, and it promotes adaptability, which makes it ideal for pregnancy, when anxiety about the unknowable can be at an all-time high. Practicing mindfulness can be as simple as approaching your daily activities with awareness and intention—for example, by simply noticing what you are doing, feeling, or thinking at any moment.

Mindfulness Basics

- Notice your breathing, particularly when you're experiencing strong emotions. Is it fast, slow, even, uneven, deep, or shallow?

- Pause and take in the sensations you're experiencing right now, the things that typically escape your attention, such as smells, sights, and touch.

- Plug into your body's physical presence. How does it feel to swallow a gulp of water? What does your body feel like against the seat of your car?

- Consider that any thoughts and emotions you are having are momentary and do not define who you are as person, or as a mother-to-be. By acknowledging that your thoughts are just thoughts, with practice you can break down and move past any negative thought patterns.

These simple mindfulness exercises will help you learn to process and react more intentionally to changes in your day-to-day life. When you feel you've gotten the hang of them, move on to the Five-Minute Reboot.

The Five-Minute Reboot

For a deeper experience of mindfulness, you might give meditation a try. Meditation is the practice of sitting quietly, often with your eyes closed, and noticing your thoughts and what your body is feeling. This basic exercise will give you a taste of what meditation is like. Use it when you're experiencing unpleasant emotions, including those of overwhelming anxiety or fear, or when you just want to connect more fully to your experience.

Step 1: Set a Timer
Set the timer for five minutes (but allow seven minutes total, which will give you time for the final step).

Step 2: Get Comfortable
Sit cross-legged on the floor, or sit in a chair with your legs hip-distance apart and your feet flat on the floor. Rest your hands on the tops of your thighs. Gently shut your eyes, or leave them open and allow your gaze to rest, unfocused, on whatever is in front of you. (Shutting your eyes helps you to turn your focus inward; leaving them open builds your ability to remain focused amid external distractions.) Notice how your body feels (for example, are there any areas that feel tight?), or simply notice the hard surface of the chair or floor beneath you.

Step 3: Focus on Your Breathing
Deepen your breathing (either through your nose, your mouth, or both, whichever comes naturally) by inhaling for a count of three and exhaling for a count of three.

Step 4: Find Your Flow
Stop counting and allow your breathing to fall into an easy rhythm. Observe the breaths as they come and go. Tune in to the rising and falling sensation in your body. Experience it from your belly to your shoulders.

Step 5: Catch and Release
Continue to observe your breathing. Random thoughts will arise (like shopping lists, work deadlines, and "what should I eat for breakfast?"). This is natural; it's just your mind and body throwing off stress. Simply catch and release these thoughts, meaning acknowledge them and then let them go.

Step 6: Relax

Simply sit. Remind yourself that there's nothing to do, fix, or change.

Step 7: Feel Gratitude

When the timer goes off, silence it and then think about something that you're grateful for—maybe it's being pregnant or having the chance to meditate. Then shift your thoughts to how your body feels—the relaxed state of your muscles and the evenness of your heartbeat and breath. Toggle between these two thoughts. When you feel ready, stand up and move forward with your day. With experience you can get a feel for how long five minutes is and do this without the set timer and the alarm going off.

MOVEMENT

Getting up and out is important at any age or stage of your life, but incorporating some sort of movement practice during pregnancy is especially beneficial, whether it's prenatal yoga, swimming, hiking, dance, or Pilates. Movement can help curb nausea in those tricky first trimester months; it can also give you the physical confidence and endurance you'll need for labor, which is—how shall I put this?—rather labor-intensive. Beyond that, taking time for movement tends to be emotionally and mentally uplifting; the simple act of taking time away from your daily responsibilities to align with your physical self can be extremely restorative.

One note: Traditional advice on exercise during pregnancy once recommended activities that keep your heart rate below 140 beats per minute. These days, heart rate limits are no longer imposed. Consult your doctor or midwife if you have concerns, but a general rule of thumb is that you can continue any activity, regardless of heart rate, if it's something you practiced before pregnancy.

Is Exercising Even OK?

There's a common (and dated) misconception that exercise isn't OK during pregnancy. In fact, your baby is protected when you exercise by the cushion of the amniotic fluid within your uterus. That said, it's best to avoid sudden jumps, stops, and high-impact exercises. The talk test is a great way to see if it might be good to slow down: If it's difficult to talk while you're working out, your heart rate might be higher than it should be.

Movement Basics

- Move for at least thirty minutes, three to five days per week.

- Make yourself known. If you're taking a class, let the instructor know you're pregnant so they can let you know of any relevant modifications.

- Go at your own pace. There's no need to overexert yourself, and don't be afraid to take a break.

- Don't up the ante. Anything you did prepregnancy is generally fine, but don't try something new and high-impact if you've never done it before. It can wait.

Maybe you're already a CrossFit fanatic or a distance runner. That's great, and you can certainly keep that up during pregnancy. But for those who have a more casual relationship with exercise, here are some of my favorite movement practices that you can incorporate now, even if you haven't already practiced them before becoming pregnant.

Walking It seems simple enough, but walking is hugely beneficial. And honestly, who said movement had to be super-complicated? Walking is a big mood-booster; it also helps improve circulation and build muscle tone.

Make sure you walk in appropriate footwear; you want your base to be well supported as you continue to gain weight.

Yoga The benefits of doing yoga feel like they were almost tailor-made for the pregnant mother: more restful sleep, decreased anxiety, back and posture strengthening, decreased nausea, and more. You can likely continue with a regular yoga practice by making a few alterations (consult with your instructor first); many women also find prenatal yoga classes to be a great, supportive mother community as well.

Pilates This recommendation surprises some people. Isn't Pilates all about strong abs? Pilates actually conditions the entire core, which includes your back, hips, and pelvic floor muscles. What's more, you actually do want to maintain some abdominal definition during pregnancy—you need those muscles to help support your growing belly.

Dance In addition to the obvious benefit of being fun and uplifting, dancing can also help pregnant mothers develop better endurance and coordination. Much like a yoga class, dancing will help you gain a better sense of your body, especially when it comes to balance. And it just feels good to move your body. Belly dancing or more rhythmic dancing is ideal.

Swimming Considered low-impact, swimming helps improve cardiovascular strength and circulation, and tones your muscles. What's more, being in the water gives a feeling of weightlessness, which you'll especially appreciate toward the end of your pregnancy. That weightlessness gives you relief and also helps ease creaky joints and muscle pain in the later months.

What's unique about these workouts is that they don't put any strain on your joints—something you'll especially appreciate while pregnant. It also allows for a strong, free range of motion, while providing support to relieve much of the weight of pregnancy that can be otherwise inhibiting.

When Enough Is Enough

Back off from your workout if you experience any of the following:

- Vaginal bleeding
- Dizziness or feeling faint
- Shortness of breath
- Headache
- Chest pain

- Muscle weakness
- Calf pain or swelling
- Contractions or preterm labor
- Fluid leaking (or gushing) from your vagina

JOURNALING

The next major self-care practice that I encourage throughout this book is writing down your thoughts, questions, concerns—any and all feelings. If you've never done this before or you worry that you won't know where to start, I've got you covered: For every month of pregnancy, I've written a series of prompts to get you started. You'll see them in sections called #writeandrelease. I hope that through the act of journaling you'll be able to create a safe, open, and therapeutic space for yourself to deposit your feelings and, in doing so, to process and release them.

Journaling Basics

Choose a medium. Whether it's a paper journal or the "Notes" app on your phone, pick what works best and what you'll stick to.

Pick the time. Maybe it's easiest right when you wake up, helping ground you for the day ahead, before anything can distract or stress you. Maybe bedtime is the perfect time for you. Or lunchtime, or before dinner. The important thing is to find that workable time and make it a habit.

Write about the bad and the good. It's easy to gripe (and important to work through challenges), but a gratitude list is a wonderful thing to keep you in touch with what's working for you right now.

Writing just one word is OK. If only one word comes out, pat yourself on the back: The practice and reflection are what's important, not how much or what you actually write.

Disconnect. Allow yourself enough time to fully detatch from your surroundings and get into your own head space—ideally, at least fifteen minutes.

Don't fret about spelling and punctuation. Again, it's not about what you write or how well you write it; it's about the process.

Don't reread. At least not right away. Putting some distance between you and your feelings helps provide perspective, and allows you to reflect with more awareness and less attachment.

By its very nature, journaling is a deeply personal practice, so there is no "right" way to approach it. Use the prompts scattered throughout this book as jumping-off points, but feel free to stray from them or circle back to things that felt particularly resonant. Like many of the tools in this book, this skill will serve you well after pregnancy too. Some research suggests that as few as three to five fifteen-minute writing sessions are enough to help people move through difficult or challenging thoughts, even some deep traumas. Through journaling, you can better understand yourself, your community, and the greater world around you—the only requirement is that you stick with it.

Through journaling you can learn to:

Find clarity. Strong emotions can be hard to understand and even hard to identify. Writing them down, we tend to bridge the gap from confusion to clarity, which puts us in better touch with both our internal and external worlds.

See yourself better. Journaling will help you see patterns that allow you to know yourself better. What types of situations or people tend to be troubling for you? What always seems to be uplifting?

Reduce stress. The cathartic element of journaling can't be overstated. When you put words to paper (or screen), it feels like a weight has been lifted; you don't have to carry all those heavy thoughts with you anymore. In turn and over time, this can significantly reduce overall anxiety.

Get better at problem solving. It's true: The more we journal, the more we open up our mental processes to both the left and right sides of the brain, which makes dealing with problems easier and more effective.

Move past personal conflicts. Writing can help you process incidents or relationships that cause you trauma or unease. The process of writing and moving through your thoughts can help you empathize with someone else's point of view—or solidify your own—which can be a strong tool for overcoming disagreements.

#writeandrelease

These writing prompts will help you access your internal compass, release your feelings, and really get to know how you're feeling at this particular time.

I love feeling _____

I am proud of myself when I _____

In crisis I _____

When I feel vulnerable I _____

NATURAL REMEDIES

Once you become pregnant, you'll notice a lot of items get added to the "do not consume" list, including many conventional medicines. This can be a tough adjustment for some, but in fact, there are many, many nondrug solutions to your ailments that are both safe and effective during pregnancy. For each month, I'll offer you several options for natural remedies that are relevant to that period—a combination of herbs, minerals, foods, and even physical treatments like acupuncture and kinesiology. Most of the remedies I'll discuss consist of nutrient-dense foods such as nettles, red raspberry, and ginger, providing similar or equal relief to some of their drug counterparts.

If you find yourself responding well to herbs, foods, and mineral supplements—or you're simply intrigued or interested—consider adding a naturopathic doctor to your birth team. Naturopathic doctors combine the wisdom of nature with the rigors of modern science. Steeped in traditional healing methods, principles, and practices, naturopathic medicine focuses on holistic, proactive prevention and comprehensive diagnosis and treatment.

Natural Remedy Basics

- **Talk with your care provider.** It's best to tell them if you're taking or considering herbs, supplements, or physical treatments. Some herbs can interact with medications, so make sure to get consent from your provider before incorporating these. That said, the remedies that I recommend in this book are mild and should complement, or certainly pose no conflicts with, any medications you might be taking.

- **Don't assume it's safe.** If you choose other remedies not found in this book, don't assume that they are safe. Herbs and plant medicine are not regulated by the FDA for safety or efficacy.

Search the label for a seal of approval from the USP (United States Pharmacopeia) or CL (Consumer-Lab.com), which indicates it has been approved by certified academic laboratories.

- **Don't overdo it.** More isn't necessarily better, and in fact could be harmful. Always follow dosing instructions.

"Natural remedy" is a sweeping term. An entire book could be written about the worldwide phenomenon across various cultures of using plants, minerals, and movement to heal during pregnancy. Most cultures have or have had an element of natural remedies, from ancient Egypt to the Greeks, Celts, Romans, and Arabs. Arguably the two best-known healing traditions are the Indian practice of Ayurveda and Chinese traditional medicine; these, in combination with my knowledge of nutrition and musculature, are the main informants to my remedy recommendations. If you're looking for more information on plant medicine, pick up Rosemary Gladstar's *Herbal Healing for Women*. Here are some of the types of natural remedies I recommend in this book.

Tinctures When herbs are soaked in water and alcohol, this extracts, preserves, and intensifies the plant's natural benefits.

Infusions The process for making infusions is more like brewing tea. Boiled water is poured over the herb and steeped for ten minutes to twenty-four hours, depending on the herb, to fully transfer its helpful properties to the liquid.

Essential oils Extracted through distillation and cold-pressing of natural ingredients, essential oils can have a profound effect on your emotional and physical state. Either inhaled or applied topically, the scent molecules trigger hormonal responses in the brain and body that promote everything from a boost in energy to a reduction in nausea.

Homeopathy Homeopathic remedies are derived from plants, minerals, and animals and are most typically found in the form of small sugar pills, ointments, gels, and drops, such as the Bach flower remedies (more on these in Chapter Five). It's possible to purchase homeopathic remedies without seeing a homeopath, but traditionally treatments are more individualized, created for the specific person and ailment. Dosing is key—homeopathy abides by the "law of minimum dose," whereby the smallest possible amount is given in order to trigger the body's natural healing ability.

Food-based supplements and compounds I generally recommend plant- or food-based supplements over those that are synthetically derived. They're easier to digest and more efficiently processed into useful nutrition. You should buy your supplements where you buy your food.

Food We'll get into the nitty-gritty of nourishment later; for now, I'll point out that food is a powerful healer as well. Eating certain foods can significantly combat discomforts.

Physical treatments Based on need, I'll recommend seeking out a professional for physical treatments, such as acupuncture, kinesiology, or massage.

NOURISHMENT

When it comes to feeding yourself during pregnancy, my usual "whatever works for you" attitude tends to diminish. Here's the thing: Cheeseburgers, burritos, pizza, cake, and all manner of delicious foods may feel satisfying in the moment, but ultimately, these foods are not serving you well. And sure, it's well known that when you're pregnant you become very, very hungry. But you also tend not to feel your best when you're pregnant. I like to try to find solutions to both of these problems at once, and the solution is always eating well, heartily, and healthfully.

Even for those women who become pregnant knowing very little about the experience, there is one aspect they have heard of and anticipate: strange cravings. If you find yourself overindulging, that's fine. But did you know that cravings are actually your body asking for something it needs nutritionally? A craving for ice cream could be your body begging for calcium or magnesium. We'll run through common cravings and some healthier options that could give your body what it really wants when we cover Month Two in Chapter Four.

Some of my clients ask me in despair: "OK, Erica, what can I eat then?" I always guide pregnant women to the anti-inflammatory diet, which is essentially a Mediterranean diet with plenty of fresh fruits, vegetables, nuts, whole grains, fish, and healthy oils. With pregnancy's inevitable ever-increasing weight, water retention, increased blood volume, and the pressure all that puts on your bones and joints, anti-inflammatory is simply the best way to go.

Nourishment Basics

- Vegetables and fruits, emphasis on the veggies and a full spectrum of color: berries, tomatoes, oranges, yellow peppers, cruciferous (cabbage-family) vegetables, and dark leafy greens.

- Carbohydrates are totally in play—just emphasize root vegetables like squashes and sweet potatoes, and whole grains, such as brown rice and quinoa.

- Good fats rich in omega-3 fatty acids help build your baby's brain! Eat salmon, sardines, avocados, ground flaxseeds, chia seeds, pumpkin seeds, and walnuts. (And maybe start that college fund while you're at it.)

- Cook with extra-virgin olive oil, butter, and ghee. Ghee, which is clarified butter with the milk residue skimmed from the top, is loaded with omega-3s and a powerful anti-inflammatory agent.

- Protein is something you'll need quite a bit more of than usual. Try to go heavy on fish before looking to red meat. When you do choose red meat, always look for organic and grass-fed options.

- Fiber is important, as pregnancy hormones tend to slow your digestive process. Flax or chia seeds can help, as can increasing your fruits and vegetables.

- Water consumption is very important, as dehydration can lead to serious health concerns during pregnancy. Fill a large water vessel and try to drink a gallon [3.8 L] by the end of each day. Infusions also count toward your goal.

- Avoid fast and processed foods; refined sugar; high-fructose corn syrup; polyunsaturated vegetable oils like safflower, sunflower, corn, canola, and soy; and partially hydrogenated oils like margarine and shortening.

- To prevent blood sugar spikes when indulging in a sweet treat, combine it with a good amount of healthy fat and fiber to slow the sugar release into your bloodstream. Dates stuffed with almond butter is a good combination.

A Sample Day

Breakfast choices: Poached eggs with sautéed greens and quinoa, scrambled eggs topped with smoked fish, avocado toast topped with a fried egg, or a protein-rich smoothie (see The Green Glory Smoothie, page 97).

Snack choices: Dates, snap peas, cooked edamame, guacamole and/or hummus with carrots.

Main meal choices: Grilled fish with dark greens (kale, spinach, collards); bright-colored root vegetable or winter squash (sweet potato, pumpkin, beet) and brown rice; broccoli, tofu, and quinoa bowl topped with avocado; or a grass-fed steak.

Dessert choices: Dried fruit; 70 percent cacao dark chocolate, yogurt with honey and granola, fruit popsicle, or chia pudding.

Smart eating almost always starts with smart shopping. You can't down an entire package of cookies if you never bought them, right? Here are some of my shopping rules for nutrition success.

Go organic. Eat organic always, or at least as often as possible. Plants and animals and the foods made with them that carry this certification have never been treated with pesticides, herbicides, fertilizers from synthetic ingredients, or sewage sludge, ionizing radiation, growth hormones, and/or antibiotics. Consult the Dirty Dozen and the Clean Fifteen for advice on the foods that should be consumed only if they're organic.

Shop locally. The easiest way to buy nutrient-rich food is to buy it in season, locally. Plus, organic food tends to be less expensive if it's bought locally. A great way to shop locally is to join a CSA (Community Supported Agriculture) program, which will provide you with a box of fresh produce weekly, biweekly, or monthly depending on their structure. Farmers' markets are another good source.

Bulk up. Buying in bulk is a cost-effective way to keep great pantry staples in the house. Plus, they tend to have fewer additives and preservatives than their packaged counterparts. You can find whole grains, nuts, legumes, and spices in the bulk aisle.

Embrace frozen. Don't have access to great fresh fruits and vegetables in your town or climate? No need to worry. Produce that's flash-frozen actually maintains all of its important nutrients from the time of freezing, making frozen a good healthy option.

Plan for leftovers. Double your batches, then freeze half in meal-size portions. That way, if you're too busy, too tired, or just not feeling it, you can reach into your freezer and thaw out something delicious. Plus, if you keep up this practice, you'll have food waiting for you when you get home with your new baby.

Mama Mantra
Pay close attention to the things that bring you joy—and make more time for them.

PART TWO

Through the Months:

Your Growing Baby

Over the next three chapters we're going to explore what you will likely experience during pregnancy as you and your baby grow and change together. I'll walk you through each stage of your baby's physical development and each stage of your own development as a mother-to-be. I'll also offer tailored guidance to help alleviate symptoms and boost your ease and comfort, and help you process the feelings and sensations associated with the new and somewhat foreign process you're going through. At the end of each month, you'll find a #getitdone list to help you stay on task with the basic things you need to do as you approach motherhood.

The nine months of your pregnancy might fly by or they could feel like they're dragging, but no matter what your perspective, symptoms, or circumstances are, I encourage you to take each day moment by moment. The guidance in the chapters ahead is designed to help you do just that. In addition to an overview of the growth and development of your baby, each month-by-month section includes suggestions for the five key areas of self-care—mindfulness, journaling, movement, natural remedies, and nourishment. They'll help you achieve optimum growth conditions for you and your baby; moreover, they'll support the greater goal of cultivating a healthy and positive outlook for yourself. Do as little or as much as feels comfortable for you; and if you find an activity especially beneficial or enjoyable, consider carrying it with you through the remaining months of your pregnancy and beyond, into motherhood.

CHAPTER FOUR

The First Trimester

———

In many ways, the first trimester is a mental game. Your body may not show physical signs of changing quite yet, but you'll certainly feel different. You'll hear your baby's heartbeat for the first time, you'll experience a shifting range of emotions—joy, nervousness, excitement—and you may have to slow down, take more breaks, and listen to your body more than you've ever had to before, as nausea, fatigue, and other early pregnancy symptoms begin to appear.

In the following sections, we'll explore the first trimester as a period of looking within yourself and taking those first mental steps in your journey toward motherhood. I like to think of this trimester as a cocooning period, in which you allow yourself the time and space to settle into your pregnancy before emerging as a fully realized (and revealed) pregnant woman in the second trimester. Whatever you feel—and especially if it's not a feeling you expected to have—treat yourself gently and take the moments and days as they come. Stay mindful of your energy levels, what you're eating, and what activities are helpful (or not). Get into the habit of taking it slow.

MONTH ONE

What's Happening?

At the beginning of this month, implantation of your fertilized egg is complete. And by the end of the month, your baby has begun to take shape and the heart has begun to beat. A potent cocktail of hormones is swirling in your body, namely:

- **Human chorionic gonadotropin (hCG)** stimulates the empty follicle that produced the egg that became your baby to continue producing estrogen and progesterone. It's the high levels of hCG in your urine or blood that produce a positive result on a pregnancy test, conclusively indicating you're pregnant.

- **Progesterone** serves many important roles throughout your pregnancy. At this stage, its most important role is building the lining of your uterus and quieting the uterine muscles, preventing contractions, so that the fertilized egg can implant safely.

- **Estrogen** stimulates your uterus to stretch and improves your overall blood flow. It also prepares your breasts for milk production by enlarging the milk ducts. It can also make both your sex drive and moods more intense, so you might find yourself more emotional (weepy, even) or sensitive than usual.

Feelings and Sensations

Although you may experience some early bloating, light nausea, or aching in your breasts, at this point most women don't know they're pregnant yet. If you've been actively trying to conceive, you may be awaiting results. Or perhaps you've just missed your period and are starting to wrap your mind around impending motherhood. No matter where you fall in this spectrum, you'll likely have a range and mix of emotions this month as you begin the emotional journey of pregnancy.

Self-Care Starters

In Month One, you might already know you're pregnant, or you might be pregnant and not know it yet. Or you might be reading this book with the hope of becoming pregnant in the near or distant future. Regardless of which of these descriptions applies to you, now is the time to begin prioritizing self-care. Here are a few easy ways you can slow down and nourish yourself—and the growing baby that might already be on the way.

Sleep

Sleep is the body's ultimate stress buster; it is the time when the body heals and restores. Aim for at least seven to nine hours a night, turn off electronic devices at least thirty minutes before bedtime, and consider getting tucked in by 10:00 P.M.

Lavender Essential Oil

Known for reducing anxiety and anger and promoting relaxation, this floral essential oil can help add ease to your day whenever you might need it. For purity, choose organic and wildcrafted oils when possible. Lavender is one of the few essential oils that can be used directly on the skin. It's also great in an aromatherapy diffuser; place it next to your bed or place a few drops on a tissue and inhale to help promote a better night's sleep. The nasal passages are a direct link to the brain.

Lemon Water

Start the day with warm lemon water (1 cup [240 ml] of water with the juice of half a lemon squeezed in). It helps promote digestion by improving your body's ability to absorb nutrients throughout the day and helping food pass through your system with ease. Swish your mouth with water afterward to protect your tooth enamel.

A Long Bath

A warm bath can recharge the body. Try one per week with two cups [510 g] of Epsom salts, a naturally occurring mineral compound of magnesium and sulfate. It will help improve blood flow and oxygenation throughout the body. Soak for at least twenty minutes and avoid water temperatures above 102°F [37°C].

Unplug

A break from your devices or social media can be a welcome change. Give yourself a few hours offline every week, and when you do, consider heading outside and giving yourself a moment to take in your surroundings.

Get a Coloring Book

Recent research has found that, similar to meditation, coloring mandalas (round frames with abstract geometric patterns) or coloring in a coloring book can promote relaxation and significantly reduce anxiety. It's a quick shortcut to a quiet mind.

#getitdone

To help you gain clarity and a little bit of direction each month, here are a few specific items to tackle that will help keep you organized.

Month One:

- Start taking a prenatal vitamin or supplementing with folate and vitamin D.

- Review your health insurance policy to see what care providers are covered. Most providers will see you at 7 to 8 weeks.

Extra, Extra

Prenatal vitamins are an excellent source of extra nutrition as your baby grows, and they can help boost vitality for both of you. If you find it hard to keep down prenatal vitamins or they give you an upset stomach, try reducing the number of supplements you take. New research shows that the most important nutrients to supplement in the first trimester are folic acid (or folate) and vitamin D.

Folate is also known as vitamin B9. It is found naturally in foods. Folic acid is the synthetic form of folate, found in supplements and added to fortified foods. Folate is preferable over folic acid to protect your baby from neural defects in the first weeks of your first trimester, before your pregnancy is confirmed. It's best to start taking it before you start trying to conceive. A study in the *Journal of Obstetrics & Gynecology* in 2014 reported that women who consumed 730 micrograms of folic acid a day before getting pregnant were 20 percent less likely to experience a miscarriage than women who didn't take a supplement.

When supplementing with folate, select the bioactive form, methylfolate (also known as L-Methylfolate or 5-MTHF). Taking the active form bypasses the problem many people have of lacking the enzyme that allows them to metabolize folate or folic acid into its active form. Discuss fine-tuning your supplement intake with your care provider, or it might be appropriate for you to do specific supplementation coupling folic acid, vitamin D, and the essential fatty acids mentioned below.

Here are a few tips for selecting supplements:

- I always recommend whole food–based vitamins; they are known to be easier on the stomach. Choose organic or GMO-free, if available.

- Make sure your chosen supplement contains the recommended 800 micrograms of L-Methylfolate or 5-MTHF.

- Supplement with essential fatty acids: ESA, DHA, and omega-3s.

- Consider boosting your usual intake of vitamin D, especially in the third trimester when baby's bones are building quickly. Ask your care provider for a recommendation; take a minimum of 1000 IU per day.

MONTH TWO

What's Happening?

Your baby has been busy. By the beginning of Month Two, her face, fingers, and toes have already started to form, and she can even flex at the elbows and wrists. Although you won't be able to feel it yet, as her muscles develop your baby will soon begin making her first movements. Her hair and finger-nails have also developed—she now has teeny fingernails. Internal organs, including the kidney, liver, and lungs, have begun to form, and your baby's heartbeat is getting stronger and more active every day. At this point, it's racing at 80 to 120 beats per minute. Your uterus has already begun to stretch to accommodate your ever-growing baby, who is about the size of a pea at the beginning of this month.

Feelings and Sensations

The hormone progesterone is running the show, and unfortunately for this part of your pregnancy, that show is typically characterized by nausea, loss of appetite, and fatigue. Progesterone is your body's natural "slow down" mechanism—and believe me, with a big change like motherhood on the

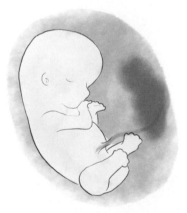

Your growing baby at the beginning of Month Two

horizon, you need it. You may find that after a deep, restful ten-plus hours of sleep, you yearn for a nap after breakfast. I've known many mothers who, almost quite literally, would have slept all day during this time if their schedules had allowed for it. Progesterone is hard at work building the lining of your uterus and uterine contractions so that your body doesn't register your growing baby as a foreign agent. It's also a strong sedative, so as I said at the beginning of this chapter, be ready to cocoon. And then some.

This month, you might be wondering where the ravenous hunger that is often associated with pregnancy might be. It's coming—but for now, progesterone is slowing down mobility in your digestive tract, while another pregnancy hormone, relaxin, is altering membranes in your intestines to make sure every last micronutrient is absorbed to help grow your baby. Pretty amazing, right? What's less amazing is that you may be feeling full and bloated, even if you haven't eaten much. And your elevated hormone levels could bring on nausea at any time of day. You might find yourself slightly more emotional as well, as increased estrogen and progesterone are often linked with moodiness and tearfulness.

You may also experience some early bleeding or light spotting. This occurs for about 25 to 40 percent of women during the first twelve weeks of pregnancy. It can be caused by implantation bleeding, which occurs about four weeks into your pregnancy as the fertilized egg attaches to your uterine wall. Hormonal changes, sex, or a vaginal exam or transvaginal ultrasound done by your obstetrician or midwife can cause it as well. Vaginal bleeding during pregnancy can be a symptom of a larger problem, so alert your doctor right away, and be prepared to give information about the amount of blood you've lost and a description of how you're feeling overall, but try not to worry too much—more often than not, even if there is light spotting during the first trimester, the pregnancy will progress totally normally.

In Vino Veritas

The American Academy of Pediatrics recommends that pregnant women not drink alcohol. However, it also acknowledges that while doctors agree on the negative effects of alcohol abuse during pregnancy, there is no evidence to prove that occasional drinking is hazardous to unborn babies. That's largely due to the fact that setting up a clinical trial in which one group of pregnant women abstains and the other drinks occasionally poses a few ethical issues.

Ultimately, the aggregate of all this advice on pregnant drinking boils down to a few simple guidelines: Every medical organization agrees that you shouldn't binge drink, drink in your first trimester, or drink more than one or two drinks once or twice a week throughout the duration of your pregnancy. Within these guidelines, most experts seem to agree, each woman may do what feels right to her. Keep in mind that there is no "safe" threshold for alcohol exposure, and effects will vary from woman to woman.

Staying Inspired: Your Self-Care in Month Two

Month Two of pregnancy can hit you like a ton of bricks—or just slide by unnoticed. Either way, it's a great time to slow down and practice treating yourself right. These self-care practices are tailored to this month, when you might need relief from stress, nausea, discomfort, and emotional sensitivity.

Mindfulness

The One-Minute Breath is an instant stress-busting mindfulness exercise that you can do anytime and anywhere, whether sitting, standing, or lying down, by simply focusing on your breath for one full minute. Here's how: Breathe gently through your nose, holding your breath for a count of four at the top of your inhalation; then slowly exhale through your mouth for another count of four. Continue breathing in this manner, letting the breath flow easily. Notice how your breath moves through your body, what it feels like to breathe in and then out. Your mind will wander, and that's just fine; don't judge it. Let your mind go in any direction it likes. Briefly notice what images or thoughts arise and then gently refocus on your breath, and notice it entering and leaving your body. Set a timer beforehand so you know when one minute has passed, or take the "one minute" less literally and do the exercise until you feel like you've hit a mini reset button.

#writeandrelease

Introspection is the focus of this month's journaling exercise, because you're at the very beginning of a huge change. Each week, or whenever you feel inspired, consider one of these questions. As you do, acknowledge what thoughts arise that prompt you to self-reflect, and write about them too.

- What do you know about your own birth?

- How does having a baby fit into your current lifestyle and future plans?

- Who are the most supportive individuals in your life?

- What do you need to make the next few months more manageable?

Movement

In the second month of your pregnancy, you may look like yourself, but you may not feel like yourself. For this reason, you may be attracted to maintaining your normal routine, doing activities that feel more prepregnant than pregnant to you. Additionally, you've probably just been hit by the first trimester mega-exhaustion and can't fathom a full workout. This month, we'll hit on both of these things by keeping up with our Planks. The Plank is a great exercise for pregnancy—it promotes proper spinal alignment and improves your posture, which reduces your chances of bad aches and pains (your nine-months-pregnant self will thank you). It's also a great workout for your glutes and hamstrings.

The Plank

To get into Plank position, first get on your hands and knees. If it's comfortable for you, keep your arms fully extended, ensuring that your shoulders, elbows, and wrists form a straight line. Otherwise, lower yourself down onto your elbows, creating a right angle with your upper arms and forearms. Your forearms will be flat on the floor and your shoulders should be over your elbows. Straighten each leg back, balancing on your toes. Make sure your buttocks aren't too low or too high—you want your body to form a straight

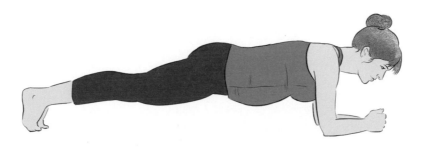

Demonstration of Plank pose

line. Also, don't hunch your shoulders or let your head hang down; your spine should be straight and neutral. Focus on lengthening your body, and hold the position for as long as is comfortable. I recommend building up to holding it for one minute.

Natural Remedies

In Month Two, you may need a few tools to help keep the nausea under control. The following natural remedies can help.

Lemon or Peppermint Essential Oil

Place three drops on a tissue and inhale deeply as soon as you feel nausea. Or diffuse a few drops in an aromatherapy diffuser; begin this as soon as you wake up in the morning.

Water

Drink eight or more glasses of water daily (ideally a full gallon [3.8 L]). It's very important to stay hydrated during pregnancy, and you're not going to believe how thirsty you get. Water helps combat first-trimester nausea, in addition to maintaining healthy amniotic fluid levels and reducing swelling. Don't wait until you feel thirsty. Dehydration can cause complications like early uterine contractions, headaches, and cramps, so it's best to get into the habit early and continue through pregnancy and postpartum, especially if you're considering breastfeeding.

Ginger

Powdered ginger in capsule form can provide nausea relief. Take up to 1 gram (1000 mg) of two to four divided doses with food daily as needed. Or try sipping Jamaican ginger beer before a meal. Reed's is my favorite—it has 17 grams (1700 mg) of fresh ginger in each bottle.

B6

This B vitamin is also known to help relieve nausea and vomiting in pregnancy. Consider taking 25 to 50 mg twice a day, in the morning and evening, to help manage your symptoms. If vomiting, add Unisom (doxylamine), an over-the-counter antihistimine. Half a tablet (12.5 mg) can help, though it may make you sleepy.

Acupressure

Acupressure is an ancient practice based on the belief that pressure can be applied to specific areas of the body to stimulate healing and well-being. This month, stimulate the pressure point in your wrist crease, which has been known to decrease nausea. Turn the palm of either hand to face you and place the first three fingers of your other hand on your inner wrist, with your ring finger at the crease in your wrist; the pressure point is just below your index finger in the channel formed by two tendons. Place your thumb there and hold with firm pressure for ten to twenty seconds. Or try Seabands, wristbands that activate these pressure points.

Balance Your Blood Sugar

Low blood sugar, particularly in the morning or just before lunch, can cause nausea. Avoid this by eating a protein- and fat-rich snack upon waking, or when you feel a wave coming on. Try hard cheese, a handful of nuts, or fruit with nut butter to even out your blood sugar.

Nourishment

In Month Two, your growing body and baby need extra micronutrients and vitamins, particularly folate (the naturally derived form of folic acid) and vitamins A and B, to help the formation of your baby's spinal cord and major organs such as the heart and lungs. But if you're battling nausea and a sensitive palate, it can be challenging to get this nourishment. Here to help are the following pregnancy-friendly recipes. If all you can keep down are white rice, crackers, and apple juice, don't stress; your digestion has slowed way down, so every last micronutrient you eat will get where it needs to go. Just eat what you can when you're up for it.

Spinach Frittata

This simple frittata is gentle on the stomach, and the eggs will help give you steady energy. Plus, it's low odor, which is helpful if you're feeling sensitive to smells, and packed with protein, folate, and vitamins B and A. It makes enough servings to last a few days, and you can eat it for any or every meal.

Serves 4

Butter, for the pan
1 tablespoon olive oil
2 medium leeks, white part only,
    sliced into rounds
6 cups [120 g] baby spinach

8 large eggs
1/4 cup [60 g] crème fraîche or
    sour cream
Salt and pepper

Place a rack in the upper third of the oven; preheat to 350°F [180°C].

Generously butter a 10-inch [25-cm] ovenproof skillet. Heat the oil over medium heat. Add the leeks and cook, stirring often, until softened, 3 to 5 minutes. Add the spinach and cook, stirring often, until softened and any liquid has evaporated, about 5 minutes.

Meanwhile, whisk the eggs and crème fraîche together until the mixture is light yellow; season with a pinch of salt and pepper. Add the egg mixture to the skillet, firmly shaking the skillet to distribute it evenly with the vegetables. Cook without stirring until the edges begin to set, about 5 minutes. Transfer to the oven and bake until the top is golden brown and the center is set, 25 to 30 minutes. Remove from the oven and allow to cool.

Ginger Root Tea

This tea helps curb nausea, stimulates your digestive system, soothes your stomach, and boosts your immune system. It keeps you hydrated during the day and can help you unwind before bed, so feel free to have it hot or refrigerate and enjoy it iced.

Serves 1 to 2

4 cups [960 ml] filtered water

2 tablespoons peeled and finely grated fresh ginger root

Juice of ¹/₂ lemon

¹/₄ teaspoon cracked black pepper

1 to 2 tablespoons honey or pure maple syrup

In a small saucepan or teapot, bring the water to a boil over high heat. Add the ginger; remove from the heat and cover. Steep for 10 to 15 minutes. Strain and add the lemon juice, black pepper, and honey. Store the tea in a 32-ounce [960-ml] mason jar to chill and enjoy later.

Looking for a bit of fizz, which can also reduce nausea? You can turn this into a switchel by adding apple cider vinegar and sparkling water. Let the tea cool, then add 2 tablespoons vinegar and chill in the fridge; add ¹/₂ cup [120 ml] sparkling water right before serving.

Navigating Loss

Loss of any kind is challenging, but if you're reading this book, the type of loss you might be most nervous about is a miscarriage. Ten to 15 percent of confirmed pregnancies (between 6 and 9 weeks) end in miscarriage, most occurring between the seventh and twelfth weeks of pregnancy. As your pregnancy progresses, the chance of having a miscarriage decreases. The vast majority of miscarriages cannot be prevented; they are random events that are not likely to recur.

Experiencing any loss can be a powerful emotional blow. Loss saps your strength, confidence, and energy, but stirs up emotions. Add an abrupt hormonal crash to your devastation, and you'll understand why it's so important to be especially compassionate with yourself at this time. The following supports can be crucial to your grieving and healing process.

- **Psychotherapy or grief counseling.** Support as you grieve is vital, and a therapist or counselor may be able to help you process your emotions during this vulnerable time. Turning to the support of a group or online community, such as Still Birthday (stillbirthday.com), can be powerfully healing.

- **Talk about it.** Everyone has a different experience, and it can be very powerful to share your story and hear that you are not alone in your feelings, particularly with other friends or family who have experienced pregnancy loss. A support group could also be helpful.

- **Let your partner in.** Communicate with your partner about your feelings and about theirs, too. It's important to stay connected and process the loss together, even if that might seem hard at first.

- **Time.** Give yourself time to heal. Grief exists on a continuum, so don't expect or force yourself to move on swiftly.

- **You're not to blame.** Remember, there is nothing you could have done to prevent this from happening. Be gentle with yourself.

#getitdone

For clarity and a bit of direction, here are a few things to tackle this month that will help keep you organized.

Month Two:

- Green up your beauty, body, and household products. (See Chapter Two for tips on how.)

- Review both your company's and your state's maternity leave policies.

- Interview and decide on a health care provider, whether it's an OB/GYN or a midwife.

MONTH THREE

What's Happening?

As you enter Month Three, the last month of your first trimester, your baby is growing rapidly. He's about 1.5 inches [4 cm] long and the size of a prune; your uterus is about the size of a grapefruit. He's active, too, moving his increasingly complex arms and legs. He can make facial expressions—including the sucking motions that will be so important once he's on the outside. Speaking of future eating habits, your baby is also developing his jaws and teeth (the latter won't typically appear until around six months after birth).

Although the major milestone is next month—when you leave the first trimester behind and enter into the second trimester—you've just hit a lesser-known but equally major milestone. Up until the beginning of this month, your baby was still in the embryo phase. With the start of Month Three, he passes into the fetal stage, during which his development is more a matter of growth and further refinement of these parts and their functions.

Feelings and Sensations

Month Three can be marked by transition for many pregnant women. Just as they say about the month of March, it can come in like a lion—with symptoms like continued nausea, fatigue, and constipation—and go out like a lamb, as symptoms subside with the onset of the second trimester (the so-called "favorite trimester"). This month, your nausea and/or morning sickness should start to fade away; you should feel a new surge of energy coming back and less lethargy, as your progesterone levels out. Your digestive tract is still at maximum-absorption levels, so you may experience constipation, and you may also experience some dizziness, as your blood vessels expand to accommodate your ever-increasing blood volume. Fun fact: In order to nourish you and your growing baby, your blood volume will double by the end of a full-term pregnancy. You might also find yourself feeling warmer than usual and may be a little sweaty when everyone else feels cool. Your basal body temperature increases slightly during the first trimester; loose clothing and cool environments can help.

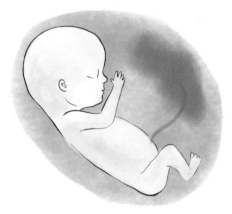

Your growing baby at the beginning of Month Three

Testing, Testing?

At various stages of your pregnancy, you'll be advised to undergo prenatal tests. Some are optional and some aren't; some test for more serious issues than others. I'll discuss them throughout Parts One and Two in the months you'll likely encounter them (Months Three, Five, Six, Eight, and Nine). Before undergoing any test, consider all the information presented to you, especially any risks, and always discuss your concerns with your care provider before proceeding. Now let's unpack the testing you may encounter in your third month.

Rh Factor At your first OB/GYN or midwife visit, blood will be tested for Rh factor compatibility. The Rh factor is a protein carried by red blood cells in approximately 85 percent of the population. If you have the protein, you're considered Rh-positive and there is no need for concern. If you lack the protein, you're among the approximately 15 percent of the population who are Rh-negative. If you're Rh-negative while your baby's blood cells—inherited from her father—are Rh-positive, your immune system may view the baby as a "foreigner" and create masses of antibodies to attack this foreigner. If her father is Rh-positive, however, there's a 50 percent chance that your baby will inherit the Rh factor from him, creating an Rh incompatibility between you and your baby. Left unchecked, this condition can threaten the health of the baby and cause hemolytic anemia in future pregnancies. Hemolytic anemia is a condition in which red blood cells are destroyed faster than the body can replace them. Prevention of the development of antibodies is the key to protecting your baby when there is Rh incompatibility. Most practitioners implement two measures. At twenty-eight weeks, if you're Rh-negative you'll be given an injection into your arm or buttocks of a substance called Rh-d immune globulin (RhoGAM) to prevent antibodies from forming. Another dose is administered within seventy-two hours after delivery if blood tests show your baby is Rh-positive. If your baby is Rh-negative, no treatment is required. The injection can be somewhat painful and the soreness can last for a couple of days, so ask your practitioner about taking a pain reliever to alleviate the discomfort. The RhoGAM injection is also administered after any genetic testing that could result in mixing of maternal and fetal blood, such as chorionic villus sampling (CVS) or amniocentesis. Vaginal bleeding or trauma during pregnancy, miscarriage, ectopic pregnancy, and abortion are the other situations where fetal blood can get into your bloodstream, so RhoGAM is given then as well. Receiving RhoGAM at these times can head off problems in future pregnancies.

Nuchal Translucency Screening Between weeks 10 and 14 you'll be offered NT screening, which looks at the folds of your baby's neck to determine whether he has Down syndrome. This test is not 100-percent accurate, but it will give you a measure of risk for your baby. Depending on the results of this test, your doctor may advise a more invasive screening, chorionic villus sampling, and a consultation with a genetic counselor.

Chorionic Villus Sampling (CVS) A sample of chorionic villi, wispy projections of placental tissue revealing your baby's genetic makeup, are taken through the cervix. This is the more invasive test to determine Down syndrome in addition to other genetic conditions, such as cystic fibrosis.

Noninvasive Prenatal Testing (NPT) At week 10 your blood can reveal plenty of information about your baby's genetic makeup. This test looks at your baby's DNA that's circulating in your bloodstream to determine her risk for various genetic disorders. This test can also determine your baby's sex, so make sure to let your doctor know in advance if you would rather be surprised.

More Than Morning Sickness

More than 70 percent of all pregnant women experience morning sickness symptoms. Unpleasant as they may be, they are not all bad, as they can be an indication that pregnancy is going well. (Rest assured, though, the absence of morning sickness doesn't mean your pregnancy isn't going well.) While many unpleasant first-trimester symptoms have faded away like a bad dream by this month of pregnancy, for some, they're going to get worse. Hyperemesis gravidarum is a condition wherein morning sickness symptoms—nausea, vomiting, and fatigue—intensify until about the twenty-week mark, when they finally subside (however, for a few women sometimes they persist even further). If you suffer from hyperemesis gravidarum, it's especially important for you to stay hydrated and well nourished. If this is difficult, your doctor may want you to receive hydration and nutrition intravenously until healthy levels are restored, or they may consider offering you medication to help combat it.

Staying Inspired: Your Self-Care in Month Three

With just one month left of your first trimester, you might be looking forward to a time when sleeping all day and seasickness on land aren't your norm. Or you might find yourself surprised by how much time has already passed. Whatever you may be dealing with, the next sections are here to help with everything from healthy meals for your (newly increasing) hunger to mindfulness remedies to see you through to the second trimester.

Mindfulness

Loving-kindness is a mindfulness practice that helps foster feelings of goodwill, kindness, and warmth for the people around you. Sounds inspiring, right? Well, it's more than just a source of inspiration. Studies show that practicing loving-kindness has incredible health benefits, including respite from illness and improved emotional intelligence. An easy way to practice loving-kindness is by making it the focus of the Five-Minute Reboot exercise (see page 55). Here's how.

Step 1

Complete Steps 1 through 4 of the Five-Minute Reboot. Once you have allowed your breath to fall into an easy rhythm, say the following phrase to yourself: "May I be happy. May I be well. May I be safe. May I be peaceful and at ease." As an aid for the first few times you do it, write down this phrase on a piece of paper and glance at it as necessary during the meditation.

Step 2

Repeat the phrase to yourself, meditating on these words until they seem to disappear. If you notice your mind wandering, focus on your breath for a few moments and then begin repeating the words again.

Step 3

Bring to mind people you feel goodwill toward, including those you know well (like family, friends, and neighbors) and those you might not know well or at all (like acquaintances or a stranger you may have passed on the street). Repeat the meditation with each person in mind, replacing the word "I" with "you."

Step 4

Turn your attention to people with whom you may be having conflict, and repeat the meditation with them in mind.

Step 5

Continue until the timer signals the end of the Five-Minute Reboot.

This version of the Five-Minute Reboot is similar to what meditation practitioners call loving-kindness meditation. Sometimes during this meditation, feelings such as anger, grief, or sadness can arise. This is natural; it can be a sign that your heart is softening, which can enable you to see what is held there, leading to increased self-awareness.

#writeandrelease

At the beginning of Month Three, having settled into your pregnancy, you may feel less nervous and more ready to surrender to joy, curiosity, and open-mindedness. With this in mind, this month's #writeandrelease exercise will focus on gratitude. Using the following prompts, reflect on what you're grateful for. (Pro tip: It doesn't have to be your pregnancy—open your thoughts to the full breadth of your daily life.) Write on the theme whenever you feel inspired, whether it's every day or just once or twice that week. As you write, acknowledge what thoughts arise that prompt you to self-reflect, and write about them too.

- In the past year, what has changed that you're thankful for?
- What experiences are you grateful for?
- What have others in your life done that you are thankful for?
- How can you continue to cultivate more gratitude in your life?

Movement

In Month Three, your energy has likely returned, which makes it easier for you to resume regular activity. As you do so, keep moderation in mind. Labor is the metabolic equivalent (in terms of energy expenditure and calories burned) of an extended, arduous workout that most women don't otherwise undertake in life—think triathlon. So building strength and muscle tone is important, but learning to listen to your body and know your limits is just as important. This month, prioritize both relaxation and activity, and you'll be very well set for the ups and downs of laboring.

Another area of focus this month is your core. Throughout your pregnancy, your abdominal muscles, also known as your "internal corset," provide important support to you and your baby. Start toning them now with Mermaid Side Bends, a simple Pilates exercise that can help minimize pregnancy-related body aches that can arise in the later months.

Mermaid Side Bends

Mermaid Side Bends strengthen your transverse abdominals (the deep muscles that wrap around your spine) and your obliques. They're great for opening up your hips and chest and giving your side a nice, deep stretch that will feel fantastic after the "cocooning" period from which you have just emerged.

Instructions: Sit cross-legged on a yoga mat. Extend your right arm out onto the yoga mat for support, forming a triangle with your torso and arm. Reach your left arm up and overhead, angling the right side of your torso closer to the mat and moving deeper into the stretch. Hold for one breath. Move as deeply into the stretch as is comfortable, breathing slowly and deeply. Hold this pose for as long as you like. Then repeat on the opposite side.

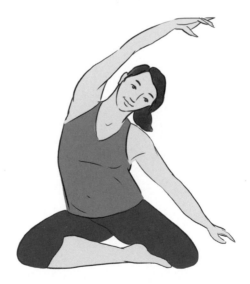

Demonstration of Mermaid Side Bends

Natural Remedies

If you are still experiencing nausea this month, refer to the natural remedies in Month Two (see page 82) and try adding a supplement of 100 to 300 mg of vitamin B6 daily. Constipation, caused by pregnancy hormones, is another common symptom of this phase of your pregnancy. Try these remedies for relief.

Fiber and Water

You'll want to make sure to get 20 to 30 grams of fiber every day (from the likes of whole grains, fruits, vegetables, and legumes). Drink plenty of water—fluids help avoid the bloating and flatulence caused by all that fiber. Be patient: The laxative effect can take three to five days to take hold. If you cannot maintain an adequate fiber intake, use 2 tablespoons of a fiber supplement, slowly increasing to up to 8 tablespoons daily as needed.

Prunes and Figs

Eating these fruits will get things moving (and provide you with an all-natural sweet fix, free from refined sugar). Keep a stash in a jar on your kitchen countertop or in a bag in your purse.

Fennel Tea

Drink fennel tea, a gentle laxative, when you first wake up to help stimulate your bowels and promote overall digestive health.

Magnesium

Also a gentle laxative, magnesium helps prevent constipation by relaxing the walls of the colon. It's especially helpful if you're under stress. A saline laxative, it increases water content, softening the stool to make for easier bowel movements. Magnesium chelate (magnesium glycinate) is gentle, can help with bowel release, and can help you sleep. Take 300 mg after food or before bed.

Nourishment

Your nourishment needs this month call for an increase in protein and zinc. These days, you'll need 75 to 100 grams of protein per day (whereas pre-pregnancy you needed only 45). Fortunately, many foods contain protein, so this is an easy need to address. Common sources of protein are meat, poultry, eggs, and dairy, plus legumes, nuts, seeds, many vegetables, and even some grains, like quinoa. Not only is protein crucial for helping your body build your baby, but it also helps stabilize your blood sugar levels, which will keep cravings under control. Zinc helps both you and your baby—you, by being a natural immune booster, and your baby, by filling his needs for protein and DNA synthesis. Sources of zinc are beef, lamb, sesame and pumpkin seeds, spinach, asparagus, and shiitake and crimini mushrooms. The following recipes will help ensure you meet your body's needs for protein and zinc this month.

....

Lentil, Sweet Potato, and Broccolini Grain Bowl

This make-ahead bowl is delicious and rich with protein and fiber. Just one cup [200 g] of lentils has around 18 grams of protein, and one sweet potato has about 2 grams in addition to vitamin A, and it is also a very good source of vitamin C, manganese, copper, vitamin B6, and phosphorus. A true superfood! Feel free to switch out the broccolini for other seasonal veggies. This dish can be served hot or at room temperature.

Serves 4 as a main meal

4 cups [960 ml] water
1 cup [200 g] green lentils, rinsed and
  drained
2 sprigs fresh thyme
Olive oil
2 whole sweet potatoes, peeled and
  cut into 1-inch [2.5-cm] pieces
1 bunch broccolini or 1 head broccoli,
  cut into bite-size florets

Sea salt and black pepper
Feta cheese (optional)

Dressing
1 teaspoon Dijon mustard
1/4 cup [60 ml] white wine vinegar
1 tablespoon fresh lemon juice
1/4 cup [60 ml] olive oil
1 teaspoon maple syrup

In a small heavy saucepan, bring the water to a boil over high heat. Add the lentils and thyme; turn the heat to low and simmer until the lentils are al dente, about 25 minutes. Drain, cool, and season to taste with olive oil; remove the thyme sprigs.

Arrange the oven racks evenly and preheat the oven to 400°F [200°C]. Toss and coat the sweet potatoes in olive oil and season with salt, then arrange on a rimmed baking sheet and roast for 15 minutes. Meanwhile, arrange the broccolini on another rimmed baking sheet and drizzle with olive oil; season with salt and pepper, and toss. Once the potatoes have roasted for 15 minutes, add the broccolini to the oven and roast both for another 15 minutes.

For the dressing: Whisk all the ingredients together in a small bowl, or shake them in a small jar until combined.

Assemble by spooning a portion of first the lentils, then the sweet potato and broccolini into a bowl. Season to taste with dressing and top with feta.

....

The Green Glory Smoothie

This creamy smoothie is fun to make and a favorite among my clients. An excellent combination of protein, fat, and fiber with a good dose of zinc, it'll help get your bowels moving if constipation is an issue, and it goes down easy any time of day. Because it is so hearty, you could even have it for dinner!

Serves 1

2 cups [40 g] raw baby spinach or kale leaves (discard the thick rib in the center of the kale leaf)

2 scoops organic grass-fed whey protein powder

1 teaspoon spirulina

2 tablespoons almond butter

2 tablespoons chia seeds

$1^3/_4$ cups [420 ml] whole milk (organic, grassfed) or nondairy milk of your choice

$1/_2$ pitted date

1 tablespoon coconut oil

$1/_4$ avocado

Place all the ingredients in a high-speed blender and blend until creamy. Drink immediately or refrigerate in a cup with a lid and give it a shake to help blend.

....

Nettle Raspberry Infusion

An herbal infusion is very much like a tea, only you use a larger quantity of herbs and steep it longer. Infusions also have a richer color and density than teas. The purpose of an herbal infusion is to nourish your body with a high dose of plant-based vitamins and minerals. For example, one cup [240 ml] of nettle tea has 5 to 10 mg of calcium, whereas a cup of nettle infusion can contain up to 500 mg of calcium.

Nettle is rich in calcium, iron, and other minerals. Super nourishing for pregnancy, nettle helps fight fatigue and acts as a diuretic, helping to reduce excess swelling. Red raspberry leaf tonifies and nourishes the uterine muscles and delivers a highly digestible form of chelated iron. The lemon balm and cinnamon add flavor and promote digestion.

It's best to make this before heading to bed, so that it's ready to drink in the morning. You can enjoy it throughout your entire pregnancy and postpartum period. Aim for at least one to three cups [240 to 720 ml] per day.

Makes 4 cups [960 ml]

¹/₄ cup [8 g] dried nettle leaves

¹/₄ cup [8 g] dried red raspberry leaves

¹/₂ cinnamon stick (optional)

4 cups [960 ml] water

Honey

Lemon

Place the nettle and raspberry leaves and cinnamon stick in a lidded 32-ounce [960-ml] wide-neck mason jar. Boil the water and pour it into the jar. Cover tightly with a lid and allow the infusion to steep for a minimum of 30 minutes and up to 8 hours (it will be inky or tawny in color). Strain after steeping and serve hot, warm, at room temperature, or iced. Add a teaspoon of honey and a squeeze of lemon juice to each cup before drinking. Keep the remaining infusion refrigerated, and discard after 36 hours.

#getitdone

For clarity and a bit of direction, here are a few things to tackle this month that will help keep you organized.

Month Three:

- Start building your baby registry.

- Start planning a babymoon (take it before week 30; after this you may feel too tired to travel).

Mama Mantra
Take it moment by moment and trust your process.

CHAPTER FIVE

The Second Trimester

Welcome to the second trimester, the celebration emoji of trimesters. Here's why women love this trimester: Nausea has abated, energy is back up (relatively), and you'll generally start to feel more yourself that you have in several months. Plus, you are adorably pregnant right now—you've got a little bump that prompts the goodwill of strangers (doors will be opened, seats will be offered, groceries will be carried), but you're not so large that you can't, say, get out of a chair unassisted.

Of course, I get it: You don't really feel back to normal. But trust me: These are the months to see friends, create community, take your childbirth and parenting classes, be active, and really get into a rhythm with your pregnancy. In the following sections, we'll break down exactly how to do that. We'll work on new mindfulness techniques, journaling, movements, and lots of incredibly nourishing and delicious recipes for your new bottomless hunger. It's going to be a lot of fun! Let's get started.

MONTH FOUR

What's Happening?

Wait a minute, what was that?! Gas? Maybe. A hungry belly-gurgle? Perhaps. Or was it your baby's first detectable movements? It can be tough to tell the difference between your normal bodily functions and the first signs of your baby's growing muscular ability, but at some point there will be no doubt what you're feeling is your baby's "quickening"—her actual movements. At this stage, she's really starting to gain mass and is roughly the size of your open palm. She's gained lots of muscle tissue, which enables her to have those stronger movements you begin to feel. In addition to detectable movements, she's also perfecting more subtle moves like yawning and sucking, which she's practicing nearly all the time. Lastly, your baby's nervous system is becoming more complex. At this point, her hearing is beginning to improve and she's able to hear your bodily functions and your voice as it reverberates on the inside.

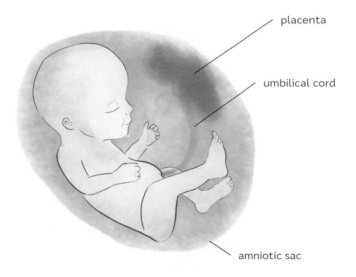

placenta

umbilical cord

amniotic sac

Your growing baby at the beginning of Month Four

Feelings and Sensations

Now that the first trimester is behind you, and hopefully the nausea as well, your symptoms will begin to manifest the more physical side of pregnancy as both you and your baby steadily grow together. If you hadn't already, by now you're decidedly showing. As your baby begins to gain mass, you may feel an aching pain in your round ligament, which is part of the support structure for your uterus. As your baby grows, the ligaments stretch, and so comes the pain, which is felt as sudden sharp spasms under the belly or groin. Your uterus is also putting pressure on the inferior vena cava, a major artery on the right side of your body. This pressure can impair circulation and can result in, I'm sorry to say, varicose veins. You might also notice that your vision is blurry. Pregnancy hormones reduce tear production, which can lead to dry eyes, irritation, and discomfort. The same hormones also cause fluid buildup in your eyes, which can lead to changes in the curvature of the eyeball, temporarily changing or degrading your vision while you're pregnant. This will self-correct after you have your baby. Lastly, you're probably feeling fairly bloated throughout this month. And you may not have anticipated it, but those inflammation-causing pregnancy hormones can also cause sinus congestion and a stuffed nose.

Staying Inspired: Your Self-Care in Month Four

Up until this point, you may have felt too tired or too unwell to really dive into the self-care practices I described (if you did manage to do them, right on!). This month, and for the rest of this trimester, your resilience will be at a high water mark—so take this time to really dig in and support yourself, while you have the energy to do so.

Getting Busy

Generally speaking, sex is totally safe during pregnancy. In fact, it is encouraged! Not only does it maintain a sense of connection with your partner, but it also can help boost your body confidence as your body grows, shifts, and changes. What's more, your libido is probably through the roof, due to an increase in estrogen and progesterone. You probably don't need me to tell you that sex is a good idea right now.

Here are a few tips and facts about sex during pregnancy:

- There's no chance of hurting your baby during sex; he's got a solid buffer, with both your healthy cervix and plenty of amniotic fluid.

- Never have oral sex if your partner has a cold sore or STD, which should be treated right away.

- Orgasms can cause Braxton Hicks contractions, which are normal and not an indication of labor.

- Spotting or slight bleeding is not typically something to be worried about, as it's caused by the normal swelling of the small blood vessels in the cervix. If you're concerned or the amount seems more than normal, ask your doctor or midwife.

- If you've been put on bed rest or are at risk of preterm labor, talk to your doctor or midwife about whether it's safe for you to have sex or orgasms.

Mindfulness

After spending the previous month exploring loving-kindness and your relationship to your community, this month we're going to bring the focus back to you. You're also going to keep building on the Five-Minute Reboot (page 55) and work on building your inner strength by adding another mantra. To begin, sit in a neutral, comfortable position with your hands resting on your lap. Maintain a neutral gaze, or if it helps you, close your eyes. Take a deep breath in for a count of four and exhale for another count of four. Settle into normal, gentle breathing, neither shallow nor deep. Instead of following your breathing or trying to escape thoughts, this time we'll repeat a mantra. Either to yourself or out loud, in a relaxing, affirming tone, say:

"I am enough, my body is strong, my baby is strong, and we are surrounded by what we need."

#writeandrelease

This month, I'd like to focus on the concept of slowing down. I encourage you to try this in areas of your life that allow for it. My three simple prompts this week will help you become aware of your usual pace, and notice where and how you can slow down and take stock to help promote more ease in each day. Slowing your pace can help reduce stress, which is so important for navigating pregnancy, labor, and motherhood—hey, and life, too.

- What part of your day feels the most busy?
- List two things you could shift to help make that time of day less busy (waking up earlier, packing a lunch for work, and so on).
- What activities help you slow down?

Movement

With nausea most likely at bay, you may find your appetite has improved, bringing with it some digestive troubles, some of which you may experience throughout your pregnancy. For that reason, Diamond pose is a great one to learn right now and keep in mind for the following six months as well. Not only does it help alleviate back pain by both stretching and strengthening your back, but it also helps stretch and strengthen your thigh muscles. It's known for easing a variety of stomach issues, including constipation, increased acidity, and gas (if you haven't experienced these just yet, at some point during pregnancy you will).

The Diamond Pose

To try Diamond pose, sit on a yoga mat with your buttocks resting on your heels. Let your palms rest on your thighs, facing up or down, and keep your head, neck, and back erect. Hold the position for a count of thirty to sixty seconds, taking in a few deep breaths. Focus on your inhalations and exhalations, and finally, taking a deep exhalation, rise up on your knees, sit back on your behind, and slowly stretch your legs outward. Take one more moment to relax, with your hands resting gently on the floor on either side of you.

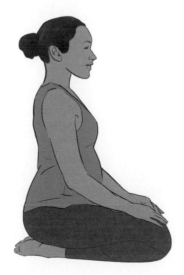

Demonstration of Diamond pose

Natural Remedies

This month you may start experiencing more of the feelings and sensations outlined earlier. What follows are effective natural remedies to help ease your more discomforting symptoms.

Varicose Veins

With more weight, more blood volume, and impaired circulation, varicose veins can become a problem. To encourage stronger circulation, use witch hazel, rubbed directly over the veins with a large cotton pad or gauze; the astringency of witch hazel will help shrink the enlarged vein and relieve the aching and throbbing. Elevate your legs at the end of the day: lie on the floor with your legs up against the wall for 5 to 10 minutes.

Stuffy Nose

Another result of increased blood flow, a chronically stuffy nose is also very common during pregnancy. Try a steamy shower before bed and a humidifier in your room for a more restful night's sleep. And when in doubt, go spicy with flavor! Horseradish, wasabi, and ginger will help clear you out—even if only temporarily.

Sore Breasts

Leafy vegetables and vitamin-rich grains can help by balancing the hormones related to breast soreness. Flaxseed oil is a helpful anti-inflammatory, so consider adding a tablespoon to oatmeal or a smoothie.

Blurry Vision

Consider natural eye drops. If you wear contacts, switch to glasses for the duration of your pregnancy. And give your eyes a rest—cut down or cut off screen time after 8:00 P.M.

Nourishment

Here's the part of the book where I get excited about calcium intake. I love talking about this, because it's such a great example of the importance of self-care during pregnancy. During these crucial months in your baby's development, he's gaining mass, muscle, and that strong skeleton that will carry him for the rest of his life. And he needs calcium—lots of it—to make that happen. If you aren't supplementing calcium or getting enough from your food, guess where he'll take it from? Your bones. This month, we'll focus on foods that support a healthy calcium intake. Remember: Helping yourself is helping your baby.

Plenty of Fish

DHA and EPA are fatty acids that are crucial to healthy brain development and memory function and even help reduce preterm birth. The best sources for both are in fish—especially wild salmon and bone-in sardines. The benefits of eating fish also outweigh any perceived risks. In a new study, consuming two to three servings of adequately cooked fish per week is recommended for pregnant women—even tuna, which pregnant women are typically told to avoid due to heavy mercury levels, as babies exposed to mercury in the womb can have brain damage and hearing and vision problems. Even if you're eating up to the recommended limit of 12 ounces [340 g] of fish per week, it's a good idea to include a supplement as part of your routine as well.

Further, by all means have some sushi. The fear concerning sushi has to do with potential bacteria or parasites, primarily salmonella, which doesn't affect pregnant women any differently than nonpregnant women. Also, most sushi fish is flash-frozen, killing parasites and microbes. There is also no scientific evidence linking sushi to birth defects or any other pregnancy abnormalities. That said, be mindful about the type of sushi you eat: Skip the vacuum-packed stuff at the grocery story or deli. Choose a high-quality, busy sushi restaurant; that way you can trust that the fish you are getting hasn't been sitting around for too long.

Farfalle with Tomatoes, Corn, Zucchini, and Ricotta

Pregnancy is all about comfort food, and this certainly is that. You may know farfalle as "bow-tie" pasta. Added bonus: The ricotta has about 300 grams of calcium.

Serves 2

½ pound [230 g] farfalle pasta

¼ cup [60 ml] olive oil, divided

1 clove garlic, finely chopped

1 cup [140 g] frozen corn, drained, or fresh corn if in season

2 small zucchinis, cut into ¼-inch [6-mm] cubes

Salt

2 cups [600 g] halved cherry tomatoes

10 large basil leaves, torn into smaller pieces

½ cup [120 g] good-quality ricotta, divided

Bring a large pot of salted water to a boil. Cook the pasta according to package directions. Drain, reserving ½ cup [120 ml] of the cooking water.

Meanwhile, heat 2 tablespoons of the olive oil in a large, high-sided skillet over low heat. Add the garlic and sauté until softened and fragrant, but not browned, 3 to 5 minutes. Increase the heat to medium and add the corn, zucchini, and 1 teaspoon of the salt. Cook for 1 to 2 minutes, then add the tomatoes and another pinch of salt. When the mixture bubbles, turn the heat down to medium-low and simmer. Let the mixture thicken without drying out.

Toss the pasta with the remaining 2 tablespoons olive oil, then add the pasta to the skillet. Stir until well combined, adding the reserved pasta water as needed to thin the sauce and prevent the pasta from sticking. Then add the basil and ¼ cup [60 ml] of the ricotta, and stir to combine. Serve with a dollop of ricotta.

Salmon Tacos with Cabbage Slaw

Have your friends over, eat flavor-packed tacos, and satisfy your DHA/EPA quota? What could be better?

Serves 4

1/2 small red cabbage, thinly sliced
1 avocado, peeled, pitted,
   and chopped
3 tablespoons fresh lime juice
1/4 cup [60 ml] extra-virgin olive oil,
   divided
Sea salt
1 pound [455 g] skin-on salmon fillet
1 teaspoon cumin

Pepper
4 corn tortillas
A bunch fresh cilantro leaves
   (optional)

Crema
1/3 cup [80 g] sour cream
2 teaspoons fresh lime juice
1/2 teaspoon finely grated lime zest

Combine the cabbage, avocado, 3 tablespoons lime juice, and 2 tablespoons of the oil in a medium bowl. Toss to combine and season to taste with salt. Set the slaw aside.

Season the salmon with the cumin and salt and pepper. Heat the remaining 2 tablespoons oil in a large nonstick skillet over medium-high heat. Add the salmon and sear each side, 4 minutes per side. Turn the heat to low, cover, and continue cooking until the salmon is opaque, about 4 more minutes. Remove from the heat and flake into a bowl.

To make the crema, combine the sour cream, 2 teaspoons lime juice, and zest in a small bowl.

To assemble each taco, heat a tortilla in a pan over a low heat for a minute until warmed through. Fill each warmed tortilla with salmon, slaw, crema, and cilantro. Serve immediately. The crema, salmon, and slaw will keep for two to three days stored in the refrigerator.

Sesame Chews

These are great grab-and-go snacks that can help stave off cravings. The sesame seeds and almond flour are both a good source of calcium (about 88 grams per teaspoon). They are also packed with magnesium, iron, phosphorus, vitamin B1, zinc, and fiber.

Makes 12 chews

1 cup [140 g] sesame seeds
1/2 cup [60 g] almond flour
3/4 cup [180 ml] honey
1 teaspoon Himalayan pink salt

1/3 cup [75 g] coconut oil, melted
1 teaspoon vanilla
2 tablespoons liquid fatty acids

Preheat the oven to 350°F [180°C]. Combine all of the ingredients in a large bowl and mix well. Scrape out the mixture onto a sheet of parchment paper and cover with another sheet. Roll out with a rolling pin or press out with your hands to form a rectangle about 1/2 in [12 mm] thick. Carefully peel off the top sheet of parchment paper and transfer the bottom sheet with the mixture to a baking sheet. Bake for 10 minutes or until golden brown. Allow to cool completely; it should still be flexible. Roll up into a log and cut into 12 chews. Store in an airtight container, in or out of the fridge.

#getitdone

For clarity and a bit of direction, here is one thing to tackle this month that will help keep you organized.

Month Four:

- Interview and choose a doula, if you're hoping to work with one. Doulas do tend to book up a few months in advance.

MONTH FIVE

What's Happening?

Your baby's nervous system has really evolved in the past month. He can hear much better now; up to this point, he may have heard only internal noises—your heartbeat, reverberations of your voice, blood circulation—but now he can hear your partner, the radio, or any other noise around you. Not only can your baby hear more clearly now, but he can also detect light. Just try shining a flashlight at your belly to see how he reacts. (Spoiler alert: He's not going to love it.) His newly refined nervous system also has a few more tricks, including his ninja grip. That's right: Your baby's senses are now developed enough for him to start reaching for his ears, nose, and umbilical cord (don't worry; at this point it can take it).

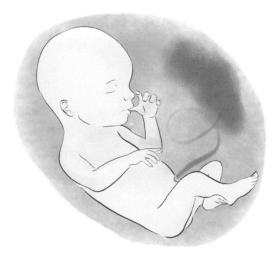

Your growing baby at the beginning of Month Five

Feelings and Sensations

If you haven't felt before that you are woman (sing it: "Wo-ma-a-a-n!"), then now is definitely your moment, as your estrogen levels are currently through the roof. If you're feeling moody, that's what's to blame—but it's also responsible if you feel generally elated as well. Estrogen's just kind of like that. This month, it's also increasing blood flow to the pelvis, which, in addition to being a nice bonus for your sex life, is also causing significant vaginal discharge. Your increased blood flow and overall volume may have you noticing another unexpected side effect: bleeding gums. Some gum sensitivity is very normal, although proper oral care is a big deal in pregnancy, so watch for signs of periodontitis (inflammation of the gums, which can lead to infection and, potentially, lost teeth), and immediately consult a dentist if things seem off. Dental health directly impacts pregnancy. For example, women with peridontitis are more at risk for preterm labor.

Finally, progesterone, that lovely pregnancy hormone that brought you bloating in the very first month, is now letting you blow off a little steam—like it or not. Burping and gas are your new normal for now, so if you aren't already comfortable doing so in front of your partner, there's really no time like the present to go there.

About 15 percent of women will develop anxiety during their pregnancy. Perinatal (meaning during pregnancy) anxiety symptoms can include the following: panic attacks, hyperventilation, excessive worry, restless sleep, and repeated thoughts or images of frightening things happening to your baby. If you experience any of this during your pregnancy, it could potentially persist into your early postpartum period, and it's important to share these feelings with your care provider and partner or doula if you're working with one. It's equally important to disclose a history of mood disorders to help navigate your postpartum emotional state. Your care provider can help refer you to a mental health provider.

Testing, Testing?

As we've discussed, not all of the possible prenatal tests are required; consider all available information, and always talk with your practitioner before proceeding. Let's consider the testing you may encounter in your fifth month.

Amniocentesis If (1) prior noninvasive prenatal testing indicates a high risk of birth defects, or (2) you have a history of genetic disorders that could be passed on to your baby, you may be considering amniocentesis. This test is generally given between fifteen and twenty weeks' gestation. An amnio can detect chromosomal abnormalities such as Down syndrome as well as neural tube defects and genetic disorders like Tay-Sachs and cystic fibrosis—all with an accuracy rate of about 99 percent. It can also tell you the sex of your baby, if you want to know it before birth. An amnio does come with a slight risk of miscarriage, but at 0.6 percent, most women consider it an acceptable risk compared to the chance to either confirm their baby is not affected by these disorders or, if one is detected, having the opportunity to decide how to proceed. If you're under age thirty-five, your insurance may not cover this test unless it's deemed medically necessary due to family history.

Staying Inspired: Your Self-Care in Month Five

At five months, you've reached the halfway point in your pregnancy, which can evoke all kinds of emotions. You may already start feeling wistful about this unique time that is passing so quickly and that you may never experience again; you may start feeling a bit of anxiety about birth or other aspects of the future; or, hey, you might just already be totally done with being pregnant and want to get it over with. All of these (and more variations!) are totally normal. This month, smack in the middle of pregnancy, we'll think about really inhabiting and taking in this time and every form our feelings take.

Mindfulness

In our exceedingly busy, active lives, there can be an emphasis, even a pressure, to go out and make things happen. We may defend this: How else would anything get done? Often we feel we must forge through something challenging alone instead of reaching to our partner, family, or community for support. As you move toward motherhood, learning to receive can be a powerful tool that will help make your transition easier. There is an immense power in developing our ability to receive—that is, our internal readiness and availability for things to happen or come to us. This is an extension of the open-mindedness we discussed way back in Chapter One— that thing that's so important for flexibility. Remember, we are better together! This month, we'll build on last month's Five-Minute Reboot (page 55) with the following mantra. Get into a comfortable position, align your breath, relax, and repeat:

"I am well in this moment, and I am open to receiving support when I need it most."

#writeandrelease

This month we'll focus on joy, an emotion that can feel fleeting or hard to locate in that busy, active life. The good news is, you can cultivate joy for yourself, and just by spending a little more time thinking about it, you might find that there is more to go around than you may have realized.

Joy feels like _____

The most significant time I felt joy was when _____

What brings me the most joy in my life is _____

Movement

This month we'll move our attention back to your core strength, ever important as you and baby hit your mass-building stride in the second trimester. By incorporating some modified Pilates exercises into your routine, you can gently reinforce those supportive abdominal muscles, asking for their help to hold up your baby (and hey, protect that sensitive lower back from potential injury!). Here's one that I love for its simplicity and also for its effectiveness.

The Upright Hundreds

The Hundreds are—excuse the pun—at the core of the Pilates method. They are essentially modified, held crunches you do on your back with your legs in tabletop position and your arms outstretched. They work wonders to strengthen the core, without the potential for back injury in many other core-building exercises. But now that you've reached the five-month mark, lying on your back for these might not be comfortable or advisable. And so I give you: the Upright Hundreds.

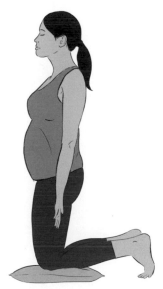

Demonstration of the Upright Hundreds

To begin, place a flat pillow on a yoga mat. Kneel on the pillow with your knees hip-distance apart. Really focus on that alignment. Keep your thigh and glute muscles active—try not to allow your hip and knee joints to rest. Your arms should be at your sides with palms facing backward. With good posture (roll your shoulders back and down, press your chest forward), begin inhaling through your nose for five arm pumps and then exhaling through your mouth for five pumps. That completes one set or cycle. Repeat this cycle nine more times for a total of 100 pumps.

Natural Remedies

This month, as you approach the halfway mark of your pregnancy, you may start experiencing more of the feelings and sensations outlined earlier in this chapter. The following natural remedies can help ease some of your more discomforting symptoms.

Bleeding Gums

Add 1 teaspoon of sea salt to a mason jar, fill it with mineral water, and keep the solution readily available by your bathroom sink. Swish a mouthful vigorously all around in your mouth and spit it out. You might also consider switching to a smaller, softer-bristled children's toothbrush, which will help you maintain your dental hygiene with less irritation to your gums. Or swish 1 tablespoon of cold-pressed sesame oil around in your mouth for ten minutes, then spit it out. Sesame oil contains high amounts of vitamin E and fatty acids to reduce inflammation and fight bacteria.

Bloating

Put a single clove in your mouth and bite down on it once to release its essential oil. Hold it in the back of your mouth until the taste subsides. Cloves can help improve your digestive function and, due to their carminative property, also expel gas. Avoid chewing on the clove. Not only are they tough to chew, but you want to maintain a slow release of the essential oil. Your salivary glands will start to really work, which also helps digestion.

Anxiety

Always talk to your care provider and partner before taking any remedies for anxiety. One possibility is the Bach flower remedies. Created by Dr. Edward Bach in the UK in 1920, these flower essences are purported to aid in navigating a wide range of emotions, particularly stress and anxiety. Anxiety for the welfare of somebody else—for example, worrying if everything will be all right with your baby—is an indication for Red Chestnut. If your thoughts won't leave you alone and you would give anything for a quiet mind, try White Chestnut. The dose is two drops at a time; for everyday use, add to a glass of water and sip at intervals. Bach flower remedies are considered safe for pregnancy; nevertheless, they are preserved in 27 percent alcohol, so it's best to dilute your chosen remedy in a glass of water and get your care provider's approval before using them. You can find Bach flower remedies at most natural markets. If you enjoy the benefits, consider seeing a homeopath for a more specialized remedy.

Nourishment

Oh hi there, cravings monster. And so it begins. Until now, you may have surprised yourself with how reasonably you've been eating. The first trimester may have been all about navigating what didn't make you feel like throwing up—and sometimes that meant eating very little. As you continue into your fifth month and squarely into the middle of your pregnancy, your hunger instincts are going to rev way, way up. This may not translate into the stereotypical pickles and ice cream—it might be all of your prepregnancy cravings, maybe even childhood favorites, with a vengeance. This month we'll continue pushing protein, which should help you stave off some of these intense food desires, and we'll also explore how cravings are your body's way of asking for what it needs.

Constant Cravings

Many women love that pregnancy can be a time to indulge in foods they may sometimes avoid for being too fattening or rich. "Hey," we rationalize, "if it's normal to gain weight during your pregnancy, I might as well dig in." And while your baby's placenta is working away, translating basically anything you feed it into the perfect sustenance for your baby, you may want to treat your own body a bit better than that and, even though it's contrary to conventional wisdom to "eat for two" during pregnancy, continue to eat well and healthfully during your pregnancy.

I like to think of cravings as your body telling you (as if through a megaphone!) what it needs, nutritionally speaking. Consult the following chart and see if substituting healthier foods for those craved foods that aren't so healthy helps keep things at bay. And hey, if you need a scoop of ice cream at 12:30 A.M., I'm not going to fault you—have at it . . . but broccoli also has tons of calcium, so it's worth at least giving it a try too.

The Craving	What's Missing?	Try Instead
Chocolate	Magnesium	Nuts, seeds, fruits, legumes
Bread, toast	Nitrogen	Protein (fish, meat, nuts, eggs, dairy)
Salty foods	Chloride	Goat milk, fish
Generally overeating	Silicon, tyrosine	Nuts, seeds, cheese, vitamin C or orange juice, red and green fruits and vegetables
Fatty, oily foods	Calcium	Dark leafy greens, legumes, cheese

The Craving	What's Missing?	Try Instead
Coffee, black tea	Phosphorus, sodium chloride, iron	Meat, fish, poultry, apple cider vinegar, eggs, nuts, red peppers, cruciferous vegetables, fermented foods, sparkling water
Sweets	Chromium, carbon, sulfur	Horseradish, fresh fruits (especially grapes), cheese, legumes, chicken, fermented foods
Premenstrual-style cravings	Zinc	Red meat (organ meats especially), seafood, root vegetables

Miso Ginger-Roasted Chicken with Vegetables

This is one of my favorite preparations for roast chicken, with an Asian-inspired bent. Plus, a roasted chicken provides a substantial amount of protein and can go a long way with leftovers. Shred leftovers into a salad, and don't throw away those bones! We'll be brewing bone broth for you to drink very, very soon.

Serves 2 to 4

1 teaspoon sea salt, divided

1 teaspoon cracked black pepper, divided

1 whole organic chicken (3$\frac{1}{2}$ pounds [1.6 kg]), rinsed and patted dry

1 tablespoon olive oil, plus more for the pan

3 tablespoons butter, at room temperature

3 tablespoons whole-grain mustard

1 tablespoon white miso paste

1 tablespoon honey

1 thumb-size piece of ginger

1 garlic clove

$\frac{1}{2}$ lemon

$\frac{1}{2}$ pound [225 g] carrots

1 small fennel bulb

1 onion

Preheat the oven to 450°F [230°C]. Use $\frac{1}{2}$ teaspoon of the salt and the black pepper to season the chicken.

Prepare a roasting pan with olive oil. Combine the butter, mustard, miso, honey, and $\frac{1}{4}$ teaspoon of pepper in a large bowl. Add the chicken and turn to coat the skin. Put the ginger, garlic, and lemon into the cavity of the chicken.

In a separate roasting pan, combine the carrots, fennel, onion, 1 tablespoon oil, remaining $\frac{1}{2}$ teaspoon salt, and remaining $\frac{1}{4}$ teaspoon pepper. Place the chicken in the oiled roasting pan and place in the oven, roast for 15 minutes, then turn down the heat to 350°F [180°C]. Put the pan of vegetables in the oven. Check the chicken occasionally and spoon the drippings over it as it cooks; turn and toss the veggies. Continue to roast until the bird is golden brown and an instant-read thermometer inserted into the meaty part of the thigh reads 155° to 165°F [70° to 75°C], 50 to 60 minutes; the chicken may need more time depending on the weight. The vegetables should be tender. Cut or carve the chicken and serve with the vegetables.

Almond Goji Macaroons

These cookies are chewy, sweet, satisfying, and packed with protein, minerals, fiber, and healthy fats—making it a nourishing sweet snack that can fill you up and help curb cravings. Almond flour–based, they are gluten free, with lots of magnesium in the crushed pumpkin seeds, fiber and antioxidants in the goji berries and coconut, energy-boosting ghee, and finally dark chocolate, with its potassium, zinc, and selenium.

Makes 12

Butter for the pan
1 cup [120 g] almond flour
1/2 cup [50 g] quick-cooking rolled oats
1/2 cup [40 g] shredded unsweetened coconut
1/4 cup [35 g] pumpkin seeds, crushed (use a blender or a mortar and pestle)
1 egg

1/2 cup [120 ml] maple syrup
1 teaspoon vanilla
1/4 cup [60 ml] melted ghee (clarified butter) or butter
1/4 cup [45 g] dark chocolate chips, or a 60 percent (or higher) bar, chopped into bits
1/4 cup [35 g] goji berries

Preheat the oven to 350°F [180°C]. Prepare a baking sheet by lining with parchment paper and buttering the parchment.

Combine the almond flour, oats, coconut, and crushed pumpkin seeds in a medium bowl. In a separate bowl, beat together the egg, maple syrup, and vanilla. Add to the dry ingredients, mixing until thoroughly combined. Stir in the melted ghee, then add the chocolate chips and goji berries. Chill the mixture in the refrigerator for 15 minutes.

Shape the macaroons into rounds and place on the prepared baking sheet. Bake for 15 minutes or until slightly golden. Remove from the oven and leave on the sheet for another 5 minutes before transferring to a rack.

MONTH SIX

What's Happening?

Your baby is about to bulk up in a big way. She starts the month at roughly one pound [455 g] and the size of a papaya fruit, and will nearly double her weight in the next four weeks. She's on a path to babyhood, and we pity the person who gets in her way! As you stretch to accommodate her, you'll notice (three-quarters of all pregnant women do) the appearance of a dark line that extends from your belly button downward: the linea nigra. Your

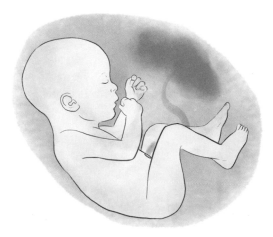

Your growing baby at the beginning of Month Six

belly button may also pop at this point as well. Your baby's face is close to being fully formed, and her hearing outside of your body continues to improve. She might even react to different music you play!

Feelings and Sensations

As you enter the last month of your second trimester, you may be starting to feel very, very pregnant. And big. You've still got a ways to go, mama, but now is the time when you might really start feeling the weight of your baby and your already quite-large uterus. The most common feeling related to your body's new size is backaches. The weight of your baby and uterus combined with the ligament-loosening hormone relaxin is a one-two punch directly into your low back. Relaxin is also relaxing the sphincter muscle at the base of your esophagus (the lower esophageal sphincter or LES) that keeps stomach acid in the stomach, which is why heartburn and acid reflux can be a major problem. Plus, as your pregnancy progresses and your belly begins to push upward, heartburn can dramatically increase. Lastly, you may be feeling faint at times, even dizzy. While a mild sense of dizziness—say, on getting up suddenly—and even clumsiness can be normal, repeated episodes may indicate that you need to take in more fluids and consider slowing down your routine to avoid falling.

Staying Inspired: Your Self-Care in Month Six

As you enter the last month of your second trimester, you will likely be feeling the physicality of your pregnancy more than you have previously. Things are certainly getting real, so we'll work on dealing with all of it in the sections that follow.

Mindfulness

Our minds can work very quickly and always seem to jump ahead to the future. As you complete your second trimester, the end of your pregnancy may already start dominating your thoughts. You may be visualizing life

Testing, Testing?

As we've discussed, not all of the possible prenatal tests are required; consider all available information, and always talk with your practitioner before proceeding.

Six Months Glucose Screen The glucose screen, which shows how your body responds to sugar, is meant to detect gestational diabetes. These days, most or all expectant mothers undergo this test. The most common test involves drinking a sugary-sweet concoction at your care provider's office, waiting an hour, then having blood drawn to test glucose levels. Some women find this drink to be quite difficult to stomach, even nauseating. (Gulcola tastes much better ice-cold, so ask if yours can be refrigerated.) If you would prefer not to inject anything, ask for a hemoglobin A1C test. If your test shows high glucose levels, you'll have to undergo a second, more involved test. You'll be asked to fast for fourteen hours, then have the drink again. Most women who take the second test are cleared, so don't fret unduly if you are required to take it again. Only about 3 to 6 percent of pregnant women get gestational diabetes.

If you're not fasting before the test, it's important to eat healthily leading up to it—you can even trigger a false positive by consuming sugary food too close to your test. Make sure to avoid food like sugary cereals or drinks the morning before your test. Try substituting healthy carbohydrates— like whole-grain, bran, or flaxseed toast.

with your baby and all the fun you'll have together, but on the whole, and in my experience with pregnant mothers, these future-leaning thoughts tend to be mostly stress-based. You may be working hard on preparing the nursery, or worrying about navigating an in-law relationship postpartum; you could be worried about how your friendships might change or what it will be like to stay at home, away from work, for several months. In this month's mindfulness exercise, we're going to work with the idea of relinquishing control. As you move toward birth and motherhood, you'll have to become comfortable with things that are beyond your control. The sooner you do, the better you will feel. This month, meditate using this mantra:

"I am gently letting go of anything that I can't control and the things I do not know."

#writeandrelease

This month, let's write about the idea of resilience. Do you believe that you possess it? Resilience is complicated. Taken very literally, it conjures elastic or something that easily bounces back to its original shape. In the emotional sphere, it can represent how you deal with trying situations, how you recover. Pregnancy and birth are significant and life-changing events—you've got to wonder how you will be on the other side of it. Using the following prompts, reflect on your resilience. My hope is that, once you do a little digging, you'll find you've got plenty of it.

When I'm struggling with doubt, I tend to _____

For me, a tough day looks like _____

I can resolve a tough day by _____

When I feel hurt by someone, I _____

_____

Movement

In your sixth month, you're really getting to know the rounder side of pregnancy—and all the aches and pains that can come from taking your growing baby with you everywhere you go. As your belly expands outward, you will particularly need strength and stretching support for your lower back. And this one is no joke: Low-back pain can be extremely debilitating, so take care of it before it becomes a problem. Try this adjusted yoga pose for a great low-back stretch.

Supported Triangle Pose

If you're familiar with yoga, you've definitely found yourself in Triangle many, many times. To avoid injury from overstretching, we're adapting Triangle to include the support of a chair. To do so, place a normal dining room chair next to you on your yoga mat. As with most yoga poses, this one is all about alignment, so be careful not to stretch yourself beyond your comfort level. Back off if it feels painful the deeper you stretch. Keep limbs and joints where they should be, and never lean into something that feels painful. Stand with your feet several feet apart (see illustration), knees soft, then pivot the foot that's closest to the chair so it's perpendicular to your other foot. With a flat back and erect posture, bend your torso toward the chair, straight from the hip, until your hand can rest gently on the chair seat. Bring your other arm straight up over your head to create a straight line from your foot to your palm. Bend the elbow of your supporting arm and lean into this stretch as much as possible without straining.

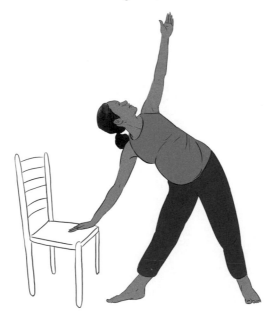

Demonstration of Supported Triangle pose

Using the chair is a great way to gauge where you are in terms of strength and flexibility. You may find that this is way too easy; in that case, I'd say to swap out the chair for a stool, a yoga block, or, if you're really up for it, the floor. If this was difficult, raise your supporting surface by adding books or a yoga block to the chair seat. Remember: None of this is one size fits all. Once you get the right height set for you, this pose will really help provide some muscular relief.

Natural Remedies

This month, as you round out your second trimester, you may start experiencing more of the feelings and sensations outlined earlier. The following natural remedies can help ease some of your more discomforting symptoms.

Backaches

These will most certainly come and go, but luckily there are some great ways to fend off a backache (without popping an over-the-counter analgesic). First, try kinesiology tape, an adhesive tape that aids and supports muscle function to provide relief from pain and discomfort. A physical therapist or kinesiologist (a health care professional who specializes in body movement) will have to apply it for you to show you how to use it properly. A second method is a maternity belt, which wraps below your belly to provide support and lift.

Heartburn

Try keeping almonds at the ready: A handful of these nuts throughout the day can help regulate acidity in the stomach due to their alkaline properties. A natural digestive enzyme—like betaine HCL, pepsin, or pancreatin—helps move digestive functions along, emptying the stomach faster to short-circuit any reflux or heartburn. Additionally, avoid coffee and fatty, spicy food, and try to wait two hours after eating before lying down. Finally, coconut oil can help neutralize stomach acid (which causes heartburn and nausea) by soothing the digestive system. Take ½ to 1 tablespoon upon waking before eating anything else.

Bodywork

This is a great month to start incorporating massage into your self-care program. If you are having a high-risk pregnancy, get approval from your midwife or OB/GYN before making an appointment. Most of the massage will take place with you lying on your side, and you'll be supported with pillows throughout. Regular massage has numerous benefits, from enhancing the function of your muscles and joints and improving your circulation and general body tone to relieving mental and physical fatigue.

Nourishment

This month we'll focus on boosting or maintaining a good iron intake. Iron is so important in pregnancy—you need 50 percent more of it right now. It's crucial for blood health and production, ensuring that both your own and your baby's supply are up to the task of bringing oxygen to all those developing organs. There are two types of iron: heme iron (found in beef, chicken, turkey, and pork) and non-heme (found in beans, tofu, spinach, and oatmeal). Heme iron is absorbed by the body best, but vegetarians can get around this by combining non-heme iron foods with foods high in vitamin C, such as broccoli, bell peppers, red cabbage, sweet potatoes, tomatoes, cantaloupe, oranges, mangoes, and strawberries—all of which are excellent sources of vitamin C. Alternatively, you can take 25 mg of vitamin C as you eat your meal, which has been shown to increase the absorption of non-heme iron fourfold. Fortified orange juice contains non-heme iron and vitamin C, which is really helpful for iron absorption.

Hey, Back Off

You've probably heard from your care provider or friends not to lie on your back for too long. The concern is that your vena cava, a large vein that runs under your uterus and brings deoxygenated blood back to your heart, can get compressed, which can potentially lead to circulatory problems. Arteries deliver oxygenated blood; veins return deoxygenated blood. Compression of this vein can indirectly affect the baby by disrupting their blood flow. My opinion? This fear is exaggerated. If you severely compress your vena cava (to the point where it could affect blood flow to your baby), guess who will also feel it? You. You'll feel dizzy, nauseous, and just plain awful. So if you wake up on your back one night (or hey, night after night) and you feel just fine, chances are your baby is fine too. When you do wake up on your back, put yourself back to sleep on your side. Prop a pillow or wedge against your lower back.

Chock-Full of Ideas

Remember last month when I severely bummed you out about healthy substitutes for cravings? Well, that's all about to change, because now I'm going to recommend chocolate. Yes, believe.

Here's why: About 3.5 ounces [100 g] of dark chocolate (70 percent cacao or higher, please!) contains over 60 percent of your daily iron intake needs. Yes, daily. Yes, chocolate. Enjoy!

Simple Bone Broth

Few things are more nourishing than a cup of warm bone broth, packed with iron, protein, collagen, gelatin, and bone-based nutrients like calcium, phosphorus, and magnesium. Bone broth is typically made from raw animal bones (chicken, beef, or goat, simmered for 24 to 48 hours, if you're interested in trying!), but I much prefer this quick and easy chicken version with aromatics. Roasting the bones cuts down on the overall cooking time, and if you happen to have just made a roast chicken you can skip the roasting and just use those bones. Enjoy bone broth on its own, like a cup of soup, or add protein (like leftover chicken) and some starch (try rice or potatoes) to make a filling meal.

Serves 2 to 4 (depending on the amount of liquid added)

2 pounds [0.9 kg] chicken bones, roasted, or bones from a roasted chicken

Filtered water to cover

1 large yellow onion, quartered

1 leek, cut into 3-inch [7.5-cm] pieces

5 celery stalks, cut into 3-inch [7.5-cm] pieces

2 carrots, peeled and halved crosswise

2 garlic cloves, unpeeled

1 tablespoon sea salt

If using raw bones, preheat the oven to 450°F [230°C]. Arrange the bones in a single layer in a roasting pan and bake until well browned, about 30 minutes.

Transfer the bones to a large stockpot. Add enough water to just cover the bones, then add the onion, leek, celery, carrots, garlic, and salt. Bring the mixture to a low boil, skimming off any fat or other particles that rise to the surface. Lower the heat to a gentle simmer. Cook for 4 to 5 hours, adding water as needed.

Strain the broth through a fine-mesh sieve into a large bowl and let cool completely. Transfer to storage containers (I prefer mason jars), cover, and refrigerate. Store the broth in the refrigerator for up to four days or in the freezer for up to six months.

Breakfast of Champions?

Believe it: Bone broth makes a delicious, filling breakfast. Try this: Poach eggs in the broth until medium-hard, about five minutes. Top with Parmesan cheese, salt, and pepper to taste.

#getitdone

For clarity and a bit of direction, here are a few things to tackle this month that will help keep you organized.

Month Six:

- Take a childbirth education class.

- Take an infant CPR class.

- Order your breast pump, if you plan to breastfeed.

- Get the facts on placenta encapsulation. The service you choose should be very experienced and have an excellent local reputation for safety and sterility.

- Get a pregnancy or body pillow to help find comfort.

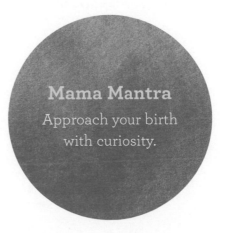

Mama Mantra

Approach your birth with curiosity.

CHAPTER SIX

The Third Trimester

Well, mama, here you are: the third and final trimester of your pregnancy. As you move into these last months, you are feeling very full. The physical side is the most obvious: You keep getting bigger and bigger as that little baby of yours bulks up in preparation for the world outside. You're also likely quite emotionally full, with strong and sometimes mixed emotions. It may feel like everything you've dealt with thus far—be it pain, elation, worry, joy, or anything else that moves you—is reaching a peak.

Anything you're experiencing is welcome, and in the coming sections, we'll explore how not only to deal with, but also to embrace, all of the physical and emotional trials you've been encountering daily. As your baby's birth approaches, you'll need more and more support both from your community and from yourself. Make time and space in your day for the advice in the coming sections—your own self-support is one of the best sources of empowerment. Let's dig in.

MONTH SEVEN

What's Happening?

You might still need a little time, but your little baby is already gearing up for his debut. Up until recently he's floated in his sac, free to take up a number of different positions, but now that space is growing scarce in there, he will start taking his position more seriously—and begin making moves toward his birth position. In fact, you may be surprised at your next ultrasound that he may already be settled in! Don't be alarmed if your baby isn't in position. As your midwife or doctor will tell you, every baby, even your own, moves at its own pace. At the beginning of Month Seven, your baby is roughly the length of a zucchini, just shy of his birth height. From here on out, he'll be adding fat deposits under his skin and filling out.

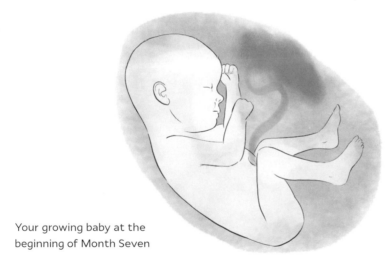

Your growing baby at the beginning of Month Seven

Feelings and Sensations

In the first month of your last trimester, new body responses related to accommodating your growing belly can arise. Stretch marks may have already begun to appear on your hips, thighs, belly, or breasts—and they may continue to appear both as you progress and postpartum. Whether or not you get stretch marks is mostly determined by genetics, but there are some comfort measures (described shortly) that you can take for skin that is stretched to its limit, and potentially feeling very itchy. Many first-time mothers also complain about pruritic urticarial papules and plaques of pregnancy (PUPPP), an uncomfortable red rash on the thighs and abdomen that can lead to hives. While your belly may be stretching to its limits, your bladder is getting cramped for space, which means you may be suffering from frequent urination, if not control issues. Your legs and ankles may also be under more strain: Leg cramps and restless leg syndrome are both very common during pregnancy. In addition to being uncomfortable—even painful—both conditions can prevent you from getting the sleep you need. You also may be experiencing swelling, known as edema, as your body is retaining a lot of fluid to support your baby.

Staying Inspired: Your Self-Care in Month Seven

After the energy and feelings of invincibility of the second trimester, the third trimester can hit like a ton of bricks. All of a sudden, you might be feeling your very real limits again. Maybe you can't walk quite as far or as quickly; maybe you're suddenly battling acid reflux, or that slight twinge in your low back has become too forceful to ignore. Whatever the feeling, this month is time to return to that caring, nonjudgmental framework we established during the first trimester. Notice and respect your individual limits; doing so will nurture you up until and through the birth.

Mindfulness

This month we'll deepen your mindfulness practice with the Body Scan, a method that brings moment-to-moment awareness to your experiences of your body. As you begin to experience some normal third trimester–related discomforts, the Body Scan can help you better identify and cope with uncomfortable sensations (also helpful during labor, but more on that

Bed (Un)rest

What is bed rest?

Increasingly referred to as "activity restriction," bed rest is a prescription by your doctor to limit your daily activity. Activity restriction can really vary in its particulars: It could mean you shouldn't go to your job site any more (but could potentially work remotely); it could mean you should limit activity to your home; it could mean you should limit activity to one floor of your house. It could (although this is rare these days) mean you are literally limited to your bed, at home or in the hospital.

What diagnoses warrant activity restriction?

Several conditions could warrant a bed rest recommendation. Here are the most common:

- **Preeclampsia**, which is pregnancy-induced hypertension (high blood pressure), is a big one. Uncontrolled preeclampsia can become eclampsia, which is essentially preeclampsia plus seizures. Preeclampsia also affects the arteries carrying blood to your placenta. If your placenta doesn't get enough blood, your baby may receive less oxygen and fewer nutrients. Pre-eclampsia is resolved by delivery, so bed rest is recommended to avoid exacerbating the condition while prolonging the pregnancy just until your baby can survive outside the womb.

- An **incompetent cervix** is pretty much what it sounds like—your cervix is having trouble staying closed and holding your baby in. In addition to bed rest, you may receive a cervical cerclage—stitches to reinforce the cervix.

- Mothers carrying **multiples** are more likely to be asked to go on bed rest simply because there are many complications associated with those pregnancies.

Are there any specific symptoms stemming from bed rest?

Bed rest tends to aggravate many typical pregnancy symptoms, like heartburn, constipation, and leg cramps. It also increases your risk of gestational diabetes. If you find yourself on very strict bed rest, you may also encounter problems like hip and back pain, muscle atrophy, bone loss, and skin irritation (bed sores). The prolonged inactivity associated with bed rest can also wreak emotional havoc, sometimes triggering bouts of depression.

What can I do about it?

Bed rest is not doled out casually or liberally, so know that if you are asked to take bed rest, it's for good reason—and there's a chance you'll be allowed back on your feet again before the birth. Move as frequently and as much as your care provider advises, and stretch in bed as often as you can remember to. Monitor what you eat (make sure it's healthy), and drink plenty of water—even more than the large amount you already were imbibing. Establish a structure for your day to keep things moving at a normal pace and feel like something is under your control. Reach out for support on message boards or from friends. Schedule plenty of visits and Skype dates. And, as always, turn to your journal—now's the time to really dig in and write it all down.

later). The Body Scan can also help you relax (and even fall asleep, which can become difficult in this trimester), connect with your baby, and discover any lingering anxiety in your body.

Try the Body Scan in a quiet, comfortable location where you can stay undisturbed for about fifteen minutes. Sit upright or lie on your side with a pillow between your knees. Your body temperature may drop during this meditation, so cover yourself with a blanket. Feel free to move into a different position at any time if this one becomes uncomfortable.

The key concept for this meditation is softening. You will locate tension and breathe into it, so as to soften it. Imagine this action as you scan your body. To begin, take two deep breaths, then bring your attention to your body. Notice how your body feels: the weight of your body on the chair, sofa, bed, or floor. Close your eyes if that's comfortable for you. Take three more deep breaths; as you take each breath, allow yourself to relax deeper and deeper.

- Notice your feet resting against the surface you're on: their weight and pressure, vibration, heat. Notice any areas of tension and release them; imagine sending your breath directly to that area of tension.

- Notice your belly. If it feels tense or tight, let it soften. Take a deep breath here. You may notice your baby begin to kick as you focus your attention here.

- Notice your chest. Is there tension? See if you can allow it to soften, breathing deeply.

- Notice your shoulders and arms. Feel any sensation: warm, cold, prickly? Breathe deeply, and let your shoulders be soft and your arms release any tension.

- Notice your hands. Are they tense? See if you can allow them to soften, staying with your breath.

- Notice your neck and throat. Let them be soft; take another deep breath.

- Now soften your jaw; let your face and facial muscles be soft.

- Then notice your whole body; be aware of your whole body as best you can. Take one more breath.

- If your eyes have been closed, when you're ready, you can open them.

- Get up gradually; as you do, continue noticing the sensations in your body.

#writeandrelease

This month we'll delve into fear. It's perfectly normal to be worried, anxious, nervous, and, yes, fearful of birth or motherhood. Most mothers have these feelings at least once and usually much more than that! And while it's normal to feel fear, it can be inhibiting and controlling, changing our experiences in ways that aren't beneficial to us or our babies. By discussing our natural fear, we can release its hold. In the prompts that follow, we'll explore your fears and empower you to let them go.

When I think of my birth, I'm most scared about _____

But I'm also confident about _____

After having my baby, I'm most nervous about _____

But I'm also confident about _____

Kicking It

Now that you've reached your third trimester, you'll want to start what's called "kick counting." Your doctor or midwife will let you know when this practice becomes crucial, but for now, just practice—and try to do this daily if you remember and have the time to spare. You can stop your daily count once you establish your baby's kick rate.

Here's how to kick count:

- Choose a time of day when your baby is most active.

- Lie on your left side or sit in a supported position with your hand on your belly.

- Check the time and see how long it takes you to feel ten movements from your baby, either kicks or flutters. Encourage your baby by drinking ice cold water or gently jiggling your belly.

- Give it 10 to 15 minutes; most babies will do ten movements before then.

By starting this counting early, you'll begin to learn more about your baby. Maybe she's a little spitfire, kicking ten times in ten minutes; maybe he's a pretty chill guy, and it takes a full two hours for him to muster ten kicks. Either way, learning your baby's patterns is the best way to find out what's normal for your baby. If there's a change in your baby's pattern or you haven't felt anything for an unusual amount of time, call your care provider and check in.

Movement

As your energy starts to wane and your body reaches capacity, comfort is the top priority. And so, without further ado, I'd like to introduce you to the "birth ball." This is essentially a traditional physiotherapy ball (exercise ball, gym ball, yoga ball); you may have seen them in use at the gym for core strengthening. For your purposes now, this ball will be used not for exercise but for ease. The birth ball is great for relieving discomfort during pregnancy and labor. It provides a firm and soft place to sit, which encourages good posture, allowing you to release your belly, and sitting on the ball instead of an ordinary chair decreases the muscle strain in your low back.

The Sit and Sway

To sit on the ball, plant your feet about shoulder-width apart and lower yourself onto it. Maintain a strong, upright posture and keep your feet wide enough to help you balance. Simply sitting like this should provide some instant relief. Begin to sway side to side or in a circle. Start by doing this movement gently; as you become more comfortable, you can begin to exaggerate your movement, stretching into it while always prioritizing balance. This is a movement that you can continue to use now, next month, and even during your labor, as it stretches muscles, releases tightness and tension, and helps give your baby more room to move into your pelvis.

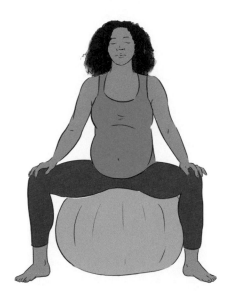

Demonstration of the Sit and Sway

The Right Ball for Your Court

Birth balls come in a range of sizes, and getting one that suits your height is important for these exercises to provide their benefits.

Here's how it breaks down:

- 55 cm: under 5'4" [1.63 m]

- 65 cm: 5'4" to 5'10" [1.63 to 1.79 m]

- 75 cm: over 5'10" [1.79 m]

If your ball fits you well, when you're seated your knees will make a right angle and your butt will be slightly higher than your knees. If that's not the case, inflate or deflate it until you get better positioning. If you feel you're between sizes, buy a larger ball and underinflate it, which will give you more stability than an overinflated smaller ball.

Natural Remedies

This month, as you move into your third trimester, you may start experiencing more of those feelings and sensations just outlined. The following natural remedies can help ease some of your more discomforting symptoms.

Stretch Marks

Although stretch marks can't be fully prevented (they're thought to be hereditary), there are some things you can do to lessen their appearance. Dry brushing is good for this: Every day, ideally in the morning, take a soft to firm body brush and brush directly on your skin over your entire body. Always brush toward your heart, as dry brushing is all about promoting circulation. There are lots of YouTube videos to show you the technique.

PUPPP

For relief from skin irritation due to PUPPP (see Feelings and Sensations, page 133), try an oatmeal and lavender compress. Combine 2 cups [200 g] of rolled oats with 1 cup [28 g] of dried lavender in a small bowl, then scoop into a small muslin sack and tie closed. Add this to a lukewarm bath, or saturate the sack with warm water in the shower and use as a compress for the affected area. This creates an oat milk that is a soothing emollient. You can use it as needed, even several times daily. For cooling relief, try aloe vera—the gel form at the drugstore is fine, but the real deal from an aloe vera plant, in addition to being pure and natural, is actually much more effective. If it doesn't improve, your health care provider may recommend a corticosteroid cream.

If your rash appears on your palms or the soles of your feet, have your care provider look at it immediately. It could be cholestasis, a liver condition in which the flow of bile is constricted. Cholestasis can cause preterm labor or breathing issues in your baby post-delivery.

Leg Cramps

Restless leg syndrome or general cramping and discomfort in the calves is very common during pregnancy. In addition to getting regular exercise and stretching, make sure you're getting enough magnesium. Legumes, nuts, whole grains, and leafy greens are all high in magnesium. If that's not doing the trick, try a natural powdered magnesium drink like Natural Vitality's Natural Calm to supplement your intake.

Hands-On Self-Care

Abhyanga massage is a powerful self-care tool from Ayurvedic medicine. The word derives from two Sanskrit words, abhy *for rub and* anga *for limb. The technique calms your nervous system, improves circulation and—a bonus for that tight skin of pregnancy—deeply moisturizes and reduces the appearance of stretch marks.*

Sesame oil
8-ounce [250-ml] squeeze bottle
Hot water in a bowl or sink

Towel or mat (that you don't
  mind getting oily)
A comfortably warm room

Add the oil to the squeeze bottle, close tightly, and warm it by submerging it in the hot water. Meanwhile, get undressed and stand on the towel or mat. Begin by massaging your scalp with your fingertips—if you don't want to apply oil to your hair, you can omit it for this portion of the massage. Work your way around your scalp to your ears and earlobes, applying firm pressure. Apply a little oil to your hands and gently but firmly work down your body until you have massaged the oil into every part you can reach. Massage or stroke from the outside to the center of your body. Use long strokes on your limbs and circular strokes over all your joints, chest, breasts, and belly. Spend extra time on areas like your belly, legs, and breasts. Take ample time to massage the soles of your feet, as this can have a particularly relaxing and soothing effect. Suds and rinse off the oil in the shower (be extra careful not to slip; use a tub mat to give the soles of your feet a secure footing). Take time in the shower to allow the oil on your hands to mix with the water from the shower and massage your face and ears. Use gentle circular strokes on your cheeks and forehead, moving out toward your ears in long stroking motions around your eyes and lips.

Nourishment

This month we'll again focus on the omegas and DHA. In the third trimester, your baby is adding more meat to her bones and more and more complexity to her brain. In fact, the highest transfer of DHA from mother to child occurs in the third trimester. Even when you're not pregnant, the fatty acids omega-3 and -6 are considered essential to brain and nerve function, and at this time it's important to make sure that you and your baby are getting enough. Supplements are helpful, but these fatty acids are also plentiful in fish, which, you know, tastes just a little better anyway.

....

Roasted Salmon Teriyaki with Spinach and Soba Noodles

Salmon is a great source for those omega-3s we're after this trimester (and all the time), and delivers many more health benefits we can use in pregnancy as well. For one, salmon is rich in protein molecules (peptides) that support joints and control inflammation and swelling, which could be helpful if you're experiencing any fluid retention or swelling in your feet or hands, or maybe even your gums. It's also rich in B and D vitamins, important for supporting a healthy pregnancy (see page 76).

Serves 2

Teriyaki sauce
1/2 cup [120 ml] tamari
1/2 tablespoon freshly grated
   ginger root
1 small garlic clove
2 tablespoons maple syrup
Juice of 1/2 lemon

2 salmon fillets, skin on
Salt and pepper
1 tablespoon olive oil
One 8-ounce [230-g] package soba
   noodles
1 generous handful baby spinach
1 teaspoon sesame oil

(continued)

Combine all the teriyaki sauce ingredients in a blender and set aside.

Preheat the oven to 450°F [230°C]. Line a large rimmed sheet pan with parchment paper. Arrange the salmon, skin side up, on the prepared pan. Season with salt and pepper and drizzle with the olive oil. Roast the salmon for 12 to 15 minutes, or until the skin crisps and the fish flakes easily when pierced with a fork.

Meanwhile, boil the soba noodles according to the package directions and drain. While still piping hot, add the spinach and sesame oil and toss to wilt the spinach. Top with the salmon and teriyaki sauce and serve.

....

Simple Chia Pudding

A food staple of the Aztecs, tiny black chia seeds pack more omega-3 fatty acids into 2 tablespoons than a 4-ounce [115-g] serving of salmon. They're also rich in fiber and protein, both of which you need at this stage. When combined with liquid, chia seeds undergo a gelatinous transformation. Combined with creamy and mineral-rich coconut milk, this pudding is a really delicious vegan treat, but feel free to use dairy if you prefer or crave it. I love this pudding for breakfast with fruit or as an after-dinner treat on its own.

Serves 2

¼ cup [45 g] chia seeds
1 teaspoon maple syrup
¾ cup [180 ml] coconut or other
 nut milk

Pinch of cinnamon
Bananas, blueberries, or coconut,
 for garnish

In a medium bowl, combine the chia seeds, maple syrup, coconut milk, and cinnamon. Stir for a couple of minutes, until very well combined and starting to thicken. Top with fruit and eat immediately, or let sit in the refrigerator for up to 48 hours; the longer it sits, the thicker it gets.

....

#getitdone

For clarity and a bit of direction, here are a few things to tackle this month that will help keep you organized.

Month Seven:

- Take a tour of your birth center or hospital.

- Order home birth supplies.

- Have a shower or blessingway, a sacred prebirth ceremony based on traditional Navajo practices (for suggestions on planning, see Resources).

- Set up your nursery.

- Wash and prep your baby's linens.

- Stock up on household basics.

- Preregister at the hospital.

- Interview and select your pediatrician.

MONTH EIGHT

What's Happening?

Practice makes perfect for your baby in Month Eight. She's getting ready for her curtain call and is very busy preparing. She's working on swallowing, breathing, sucking, and—as I'm sure you're well aware—kicking. Her body is also preparing for the big shift—in particular, her digestive system, which is just finishing up its development in anticipation of feeding by mouth. Baby's sleep cycles are aligning to her future cycles as a newborn, as well. This month she'll sleep for a thirty-minute stretch, wake, move a bit (as much as she can), then go back down.

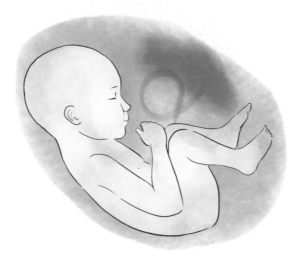

Your growing baby at the beginning of Month Eight

Feelings and Sensations

Tingling, blurring, fuzziness—just a few of the very vague-yet-acute feelings you might be experiencing this month. For one thing, pregnancy swelling is putting pressure on almost every part of your body—even, it seems, your wrists. You may develop full-blown carpal tunnel syndrome, or just experience a milder (and, not to make light of it, nagging and annoying) tingling sensation in your wrist. The same hormones that cause the swelling that can lead to carpal tunnel—and the swelling that you may be experiencing in your ankles and feet—can also cause blurred vision, dry eyes, and even floaters. (Note: If dimming, spots, and floaters last two hours or more, notify your care provider.) Also, your vision might not be the only thing increasingly fuzzy these days. You may be experiencing what's often cheekily (if cloyingly) called "baby brain." So yeah, you may have forgotten your keys or why you walked into a room; you may have left the burner on or, hey, even missed your house when going home. Forgetfulness is extremely common during pregnancy and, as with other lapses, perhaps an indication to slow down, put a little less on your to-do list, and try and get some rest. Finally, thanks to all that extra estrogen in your system, your melanin production is at an all-time high; you've probably noticed that your nipples have darkened as a result. This hormonal increase can also cause melasma, dark patches on the face. These patches may lighten or go away after pregnancy, but there are some things you can do to lessen their appearance in the meantime (see the following Natural Remedies section).

Testing, Testing?

As we've discussed, not all of the possible prenatal tests are required; consider all available information, and always talk with your practitioner before proceeding. Let's look at the testing you may encounter in your eighth month.

Group B Strep (GBS) A GBS tests for a bacteria commonly present in your digestive tract, which can crop up in the vagina or rectum. The test is fairly noninvasive—a quick swab of the vagina—but the treatment will demand that you receive intravenous antibiotics as a precaution during labor. GBS can pass to your baby during a vaginal birth, and although most babies do just fine fighting the infection, some can become very ill, running a fever, with difficulty feeding or regulating their body temperature. Though rare, it can be dangerous. It's possible to refuse these prophylactic antibiotics outside of a hospital environment and under the care of a midwife. If you do have IV antibiotics, consider probiotics for both you and your baby to repopulate the gut flora.

Staying Inspired: Your Self-Care in Month Eight

As your belly grows, your body aches, your baby kicks, and many other symptoms start to creep in, you may need some serious help staying inspired. Hang in there, mama! While many of you may still be doing just fine, others of you are at the end of your rope. For some, the last months of pregnancy can be an eternity. And yet, you may also have some anticipatory nostalgia for this time and this connection with your baby. Whatever is in the forefront for you, we'll support you through it in the coming sections. Let's focus on dealing with some symptoms and getting you what you need so that you can focus on soaking in these last moments of pregnancy positively.

Mindfulness

This month we'll combine what we worked on last month—the Body Scan—with what we learned way back in Month Four, the loving-kindness meditation. Yes, it's time to send that powerful, incredible body of yours some love. To try this month's meditation, we'll start out with the Body Scan prep. If you don't have a full fifteen minutes to spare, lead into this meditation using our Five-Minute Reboot (page 55). Another note: If you're having trouble visualizing the love and kindness, assign it a color. This can be really helpful. Pink, orange, or vibrant yellow tones can be especially effective.

Once you've relaxed into your meditation, follow this path to sending love and kindness. Spend a significant amount of time with each point and really feel the support you're sending to each part of your body.

- Send love to your feet.

- Send love to your belly; pause here and send love to your baby.

- Send love to your chest.

- Send love to your shoulders and arms.

- Send love to your hands.

- Send love to your neck and throat.

- Send love throughout your face.

- Notice your whole body present, filled with your own love.

Movement

This month, as your baby's growth surges and the amount of extra space she has to move in within your uterus begins to disappear, let's look into movements to help encourage her into an optimal birth position. As she begins to enter the pelvic brim (or pelvic inlet) next month, your baby's position will become more or less final, and an optimal position will help prevent the risk of a breech birth and can set you up for an easier labor. What is the optimal position for your baby? Positioned head down, chin tucked in, with the back of her head facing slightly toward the front of your belly. This makes for an easier delivery, as the smallest diameter of your baby's head engages with your vagina and perineum.

There are several things you can do to encourage a great birth position—for one, don't recline in deep-seated chairs or couches. Try sitting on a birth ball, hips higher than your knees. To relax, try leaning over the ball. Finally, one of the best things you can do to help your baby into positions are pelvic tilts, which really are pretty magical. Pelvic tilts help strengthen your abs, relieve back pain, and ease delivery by helping to get your baby into the best position. They're also very simple and quick to do, so you can pop into this exercise wherever or whenever the motivation strikes. Right before bed can be a great time to release the strain of the day.

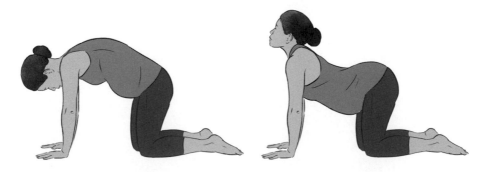

Demonstration of pelvic tilt

Pelvic Tilt

To do the pelvic tilt, start by getting onto your hands and knees on a yoga mat. Make sure you've properly aligned yourself: hips above knees, shoulders above wrists. If you've been having wrist trouble, make your hands into fists by holding a rolled-up towel or washcloth, placing your knuckles down onto the mat. Inhale deeply and as you do, arch your back toward the floor, tilting your tailbone up and turning your face up to the ceiling. Then slowly and gently exhale, rounding your spine, tucking your tailbone, and dropping the crown of your head toward the floor. As you do, add a Kegel exercise: engage your pelvic floor muscles by squeezing your vaginal muscles to the count of three and then releasing them to the count of three. Repeat with every breath as needed—I recommend eight to ten of each complete breath cycle. In between tilts, feel free to crawl forward and back or in a circle, stretching your arms and legs long as you go. Crawling is also associated with encouraging optimal fetal positioning. Try to shift between pelvic tilting and crawling for at least ten minutes per day.

#writeandrelease

This month let's reflect on the theme of change. You've already experienced so much, and no doubt will continue to through your pregnancy, your baby's birth, and your motherhood. This month, as you approach the culmination of pregnancy and are on the cusp of new motherhood, your relationship to change—and how you cope with it—is important for your well-being.

- What has changed in the way you relate to others?

- What has changed in the way you see yourself?

- Is there a change that surprised you or that you didn't expect?

Natural Remedies

With two months to go, you may start experiencing more of those feelings and sensations outlined earlier. What follows are some helpful natural remedies to ease some of your more discomforting symptoms.

Melasma

Aloe vera gel can help reduce the appearance of discoloration due to melasma. Apply generously before bed and rinse it off in the morning. Additionally, you'll want to use a heavy broad-spectrum sunblock that protects your skin from both UVA and UVB rays. A sunblock with zinc oxide or titanium dioxide is preferable to a conventional chemical sunscreen. And of course, a great wide-brimmed hat is always helpful.

Aching Joints

Give your joints a rest by eating foods that help decrease fluid retention and inflammation. Dark leafy greens are the best, and parsley, cilantro, ginger, cabbage, lemon, and garlic are also very effective. Cut down on salt, sugar, and fat, and make sure you're drinking plenty of water to keep your system hydrated and to support your body's cleansing and elimination system. Finally, get yourself fitted for a maternity bra; a proper fit can take pressure off of your median nerve—which runs from beneath your collarbone through your shoulder (under your bra strap) and down your inner arm—and help relieve some of the pain.

Nourishment

This month we'll tap into iron, protein, and calcium. You're already aware of the benefits of iron and protein, so let's talk calcium. Its absorption kicks into high gear in your last trimester. Calcium is needed to help develop your baby's teeth and bones, and build the nervous system and muscles. Milk, yogurt, and other dairy products are primary sources of calcium, as well as sardines, almonds, and leafy greens. The recipe this month delivers all three of these nutrients.

Lamb Meatballs with Cucumber-Yogurt Salad

Lamb meat is a high-quality protein source, containing all of the essential amino acids. It's also a rich source of iron. Try these meatballs accompanied with a big green salad, preferably arugula. The creamy cucumber-yogurt salad is calcium-rich and pairs well with the meatballs, which also have some feta cheese tucked in. You can eat it on its own or pair it with whole-grain pita bread.

Makes 12 meatballs

Cucumber-Yogurt Salad
1 Persian cucumber (a smaller type)
1 cup [240 ml] plain whole yogurt
3 tablespoons finely chopped
  fresh dill
1 tablespoon lemon juice
Coarse sea salt
Whole-grain pita bread (optional)

Meatballs
1 small garlic clove, minced
3 tablespoons chopped parsley
1 teaspoon table salt
1 pound [455 g] ground lamb
1 large egg
Zest of $1/2$ lemon
$1/2$ cup [30 g] breadcrumbs, fresh or
  dried, such as panko
$1/4$ cup [30 g] crumbled feta cheese
2 tablespoons tomato paste
Pinch of red pepper flakes
2 tablespoons olive oil

To make the salad, peel the cucumber and cut in half lengthwise. Scrape out the seeds with a spoon. Slice the cucumber halves into very thin half-moons. Combine them with the yogurt, dill, lemon juice, and salt to taste in a bowl and chill for at least 30 minutes while you make the meatballs.

To make the meatballs, pulse the garlic, parsley, and salt in a food processor, scraping down the sides as needed, until finely chopped.

Add the lamb, egg, lemon zest, breadcrumbs, feta, tomato paste, and red pepper flakes, and mix with a wooden spoon until evenly combined. Form the meatball mixture into $1^1/2$-inch [4-cm] balls.

Oil a baking pan with the olive oil and add the meatballs, spaced evenly. Cook, turning once or twice, until the meatballs are well browned, 5 to 7 minutes. Serve the meatballs hot with the cucumber-yogurt salad and pita bread.

#getitdone

For clarity and a bit of direction, here are a few things to tackle this month that will help keep you organized.

Month Eight:

- Solidify your birth preferences. (Consult Chapter Seven, page 168, Chapter Eight, page 180 and Resources, page 401, for direction.)

- Pack your hospital bag.

- Make your labor playlist or pick out your labor sounds.

- Get fitted for a nursing bra and pumping bra.

- Purchase and install a new baby's car seat in your car.

- Begin to practice self-massage and other labor relaxation methods.

MONTH NINE

What's Happening?

Your baby is almost ready to emerge! He's continuing to bulk up more and more—he'll likely gain an additional pound [455 g] in this last month of gestation. If he hasn't already, he'll also likely get into birth position now (if not, there are exercises and acupuncture to help encourage him). As your baby starts resembling a newborn on the inside, he's also starting to behave like one. He's certainly active (when he's awake!), but with limited room, his movements feel less like jabs and kicks and more like rolls and wiggles.

Feelings and Sensations

In your final month of pregnancy, you might be feeling a range of things: very ready to stop being pregnant, a little anxious about what's to come, or even melancholy to see this unique time draw to a close. Your mind might be racing, and that—in addition to aches, heartburn, snoring, congestion, and difficulty finding a comfortable position—can cause sleeplessness in the final weeks of pregnancy. What's more, some women deal with migraine pain, which can be caused by anything from hormones to poor hydration. Sciatica is also something many women deal with in the final stages of pregnancy. You'll definitely know it if you have it: a sharp pain that shoots from your buttocks down your legs. Finally, pregnancy can bring some surprising changes to your skin as well. Earlier you may have experienced some hormone-related acne, or you may have some new moles to keep track of.

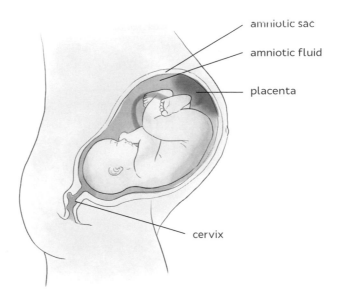

amniotic sac

amniotic fluid

placenta

cervix

Your growing baby at the beginning of Month Nine

Heads Up

What does breech mean?

A breech presentation basically means that, as you're approaching your due date, your baby has her head at the top of your uterus and her lower body at your cervix. Breech is not wrong; it's just that the headfirst position is so much more common (around 96 percent of full-term babies in the United States present this way), is considered a safer presentation for delivery, and makes for an easier labor.

There are three types of breech: a frank breech means your baby's buttocks are against the cervix; a complete breech means your baby's feet and buttocks are pushed against the cervix; a footling breech means one or both feet are against the cervix.

Is it serious?

That depends. If your baby is still breech by D-Day, she could still be delivered vaginally, or your practitioner may advise a c-section. This depends on your care provider (OB/GYN or midwife), their training and experience with breech births, and whether they generally elect to perform them. The specific position and size of your baby can also dictate your options. Breech births can be a more complicated delivery, so typically only a handful of OB/GYNs are able to accommodate them. If your care provider can't or won't perform a vaginal breech birth, it might be worth doing more research and seeing who specializes in these in your area.

What can I do?

A breech position is very common during the first and second trimesters, since there is lots of amniotic fluid and room in your uterus for your baby to move around, but most babies will flip and settle into a normal presentation by thirty-six weeks. If your baby hasn't flipped by the eighth month, your doctor will probably advise you to put a c-section on the calendar (although many mothers choose not to schedule a c-section before they actually go into labor, to avoid an early breech birth). That said, there are many things you can do to help shift your breech baby into the head-down position, including the following:

- **External cephalic rotation (ECR)** This procedure is also referred to as an external cephalic version (ECV). In both cases, your doctor will attempt to manually, externally rotate your baby into the correct birth position. This procedure can be effective, but be warned: It is painful. You will be closely monitored for possible fetal distress, if this is done in the hospital.

- **Moxibustion** A traditional Chinese therapy used in conjunction with acupuncture, moxibustion is an extremely safe way to encourage a baby to flip into the proper position. Dried mugwort is rolled into a cylinder and burned near the appropriate acupuncture point, warming the skin. A 2001 study found that moxibustion was successful in turning 73 percent of breech babies.

- **Spinning Babies** Developed by a midwife, the Spinning Babies technique involves stretching and positioning exercises you can do to encourage your baby to move into the head-down birthing position. Even if your baby isn't breech, these techniques are said to promote an easier birth. Read more at SpinningBabies.com.

Testing, Testing?

As we've discussed, not all of the possible prenatal tests are required; consider all available information, and always talk with your practitioner before proceeding. Let's look at the testing you may encounter in your ninth month.

Nonstress Test If you pass your due date, your doctor or midwife will probably bring up the nonstress test. This is a noninvasive (and not at all scary) twenty- to sixty-minute procedure: They'll strap a fetal monitoring belt to your belly to monitor your baby's heart rate, first when she's sleeping and then when she's moving around. They'll also be recording contractions. Make sure you eat before your test, and bring food and drink with you in case you are stuck in the waiting room. If the baby isn't "reactive" during the test, don't panic; she may just be asleep. If something is wrong, your care provider may suggest an induction. Like all tests, you can discuss with your care provider whether it is appropriate for you and your baby.

Nip It in the Bud

Flat or inverted nipples can make breastfeeding more challenging and potentially painful. It's a good idea to check your nipples in advance of your baby's first day of life (and potential first attempts at feeding), so that you can get techniques or nipple guards ready in anticipation. To check if your nipples are indeed flat or inverted, flip to page 349 for a few simple techniques for testing. You can also ask your doctor or mid-wife to have a look.

If it turns out that your nipples are flat or inverted and you are hoping to breastfeed, purchase a pair of breast shells—there are a few different makes and models (for example, TheraShells by the breast pump maker Medela) that help with everting nipples (that is, reversing inverted nipples so they protrude) as well as protecting sore nipples, collecting leakage, and so on. Wearing these during the day is very discreet and can help evert your nipple in preparation for breastfeeding.

Staying Inspired: Your Self-Care in Month Nine

It's all coming together now! Birth is on the horizon, which brings many conflicting emotions. You, your baby, your partner, and your community have all been building toward this moment—if you feel daunted or anxious, that should be no surprise. This month is also characterized by the seemingly endless waiting. When will baby arrive? is almost as popular a question as how at this point. In the coming sections, we'll look at ways to calm those nerves, nurture your spirit, and empower you for labor. You can do it!

Mindfulness

This month we'll move back to our Five-Minute Reboot and incorporate a new month-appropriate mantra. That said, if the Body Scan is really working for you, by all means continue to practice it. Now that you're in the final weeks of pregnancy, my hope is that you've significantly slowed down your routine. If that's the case and you've been enjoying the Body Scan, I would try to start the day with this new mantra, then end it with a Body Scan.

This month, the final month of your pregnancy, I'd like you to focus on occupying the present moment. During these final weeks, you may find yourself caught up in the calendar, watching the days and anticipating your baby's arrival. Keep in mind that due dates are not exact and that new mothers tend to deliver a few days to as much as a week or more later than predicted. Take this time to drink in your soon-to-be ending pregnancy and the transformative journey you've been on with your baby. Enjoy the peace and live in this moment.

To practice this meditation, unwind using the beginning of the Five-Minute Reboot (page 55). Once settled, gently relax your breathing and, turning away from that awareness, repeat the following mantra, whether aloud or inside and to yourself:

"I trust my body and my baby. You will come when you are ready, and I will be ready to receive you."

#writeandrelease

We all have or have had mothers. It's a complicated and dynamic role, one that carries many emotions (good, bad, and ugly) for many people. As you move into this role yourself, it's a great idea to reflect on what mothering means to you. Try to internalize these prompts as you acknowledge the past and also visualize your future.

- What does mothering mean to you?

- What qualities do you admire in how you were mothered or parented?

- What kind of mother do you see yourself becoming?

Movement

During your final month of pregnancy, you'll be at your absolute biggest, which means you'll also feel your most uncomfortable and encumbered. This month we won't ask you to try any new yoga or Pilates poses. That said, we do want you to keep active and not fall into stagnancy in this final period! Rather, I would like to encourage good circulation and a fair amount of cardiovascular work, and even to prompt that little baby of yours to initiate labor. For all these reasons, I recommend taking a walk.

Unless you're already engaged in a regular exercise routine that you love, this month I want you to just walk, aiming for one to three miles every day. Take it easy and slow—we aren't looking for your heart rate to soar or for you to reach any land-speed record. If you like a musical accompaniment or audiobook, throw on a long podcast or recording and just walk; maybe even take a light hike somewhere scenic. Walking can help encourage gravity and draw your baby down into your pelvis, adding pressure on your cervix to prime it for labor. It can also help labor progress if you've already felt some contractions. If walking is not your thing, do whatever works to keep you moving, but, especially in Month Nine, if it's too much, stop. No matter what. (I've even heard some women stop on a park bench and call their partners to come pick them up if they're too far from home to walk back. Seriously— there's no shame.) Make sure you get more rest than exercise this month.

Natural Remedies

As you move into your final month of pregnancy, you may start experiencing more of those feelings and sensations outlined earlier. The following natural remedies can help ease some of your more discomforting symptoms. This month, consider starting a labor prep regimen, like the one I recommend in the Resources section (page 428), to prepare your body.

Severe Headache and Migraine

First and foremost, make sure you're drinking enough water. Again, I try to aim for one gallon [3.8 L] daily, and at this stage, that's what you need as well. A shot of espresso is also helpful; if you're limiting the rest of your daily caffeine intake, one shot is perfectly safe. Finally, at this stage of your pregnancy, your posture may be severely compromised, which puts strain on your neck and skull, resulting in a ceaseless tension headache. Acupuncture is a really effective way to deal with those symptoms.

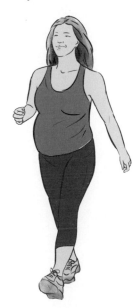

Demonstration of Month Nine
movement

Sleeplessness

Babies do really well with sleep routines—and actually, so do adults. Try winding yourself down before bed with a warm bath, a book, or time with your journal and white noise. Cut off your caffeine intake by 2:00 P.M., and avoid electronic screens in the last hour before bedtime; avoid eating for at least two hours before. Additionally, an essential oil blend inhaled directly or diffused can be helpful, as can chamomile tea. Finally, WishGarden Herbs' sleep tincture Sleepy Nights for Pregnancy is very effective—follow the bottle's directions.

Bodywork

I'm mentioning massage again because it's a beneficial and uplifting way to fill your days. While you wait for your baby, consider getting a weekly or biweekly massage; this can help your body loosen and prepare for labor, and releases some of those feel-good endorphins. It can also help you sleep and keep headaches at bay.

....

Sleep Aid Oil

This is a great oil blend to aid sleep, from my friend and aromatherapist Hope Gillerman.

Makes about ¹/₈ ounce

1-ounce [30-ml] amber glass bottle with a reducer (an inner cap that limits the output to drops)

4 drops spikenard oil
8 drops lavender oil
45 drops mandarin orange oil

Place all the oils in the glass bottle and gently swirl to mix.

Place 2 or 3 drops of the blend on a tissue and inhale deeply for 10 breaths. This is great right before bed. Or add 10 drops to a diffuser in your bedroom.

....

Nourishment

As you are in your final weeks of pregnancy, let's shift our focus from the pregnancy-specific nutritional needs we've been working with to your needs as a new mother. In the first weeks postpartum, you'll need food that's nutrient dense, quick to prepare, and easy to digest. The following dishes are two favorites that I frequently prepare for new mothers postpartum.

. . . .

Sweet Potato, Lentil, and Ginger Soup

This twenty-minute soup is fiber-rich and soothing. During pregnancy and after birth, your intestinal muscle capacity is reduced, and remains so during the first two to three months postpartum. Adding more fiber to your diet will help shift that sluggishness and keep things moving. Make a batch or two and freeze it.

Serves 4

1 tablespoon organic coconut oil

2 tablespoons grated or finely diced fresh turmeric root

4 tablespoons grated or finely diced ginger root

1 cup [200 g] red lentils, rinsed and picked through

5 garnet yams, peeled and roughly chopped

6 cups [1.4 L] organic chicken or vegetable stock

¼ cup [60 ml] organic coconut milk

1 bunch fresh cilantro, finely chopped

1 teaspoon salt

Black pepper

Melt the coconut oil in a heavy medium pot or Dutch oven over medium heat. Add the turmeric, ginger, and lentils. Sauté for 3 to 5 minutes, until fragrant, then add the yams. Toss until the yams are coated and slightly caramelized, 3 to 5 minutes.

Pour in the stock and bring to a boil. Turn down the heat and simmer uncovered until the lentils and yams are tender. Remove from the heat, then mix in the coconut milk and cilantro. Season with the salt and pepper to taste and serve.

. . . .

Soaked Supergrain Porridge

This porridge is also high in fiber, which will help keep things moving postpartum. Make a big pot in the evening (it needs to soak overnight) and eat it for breakfast for several days. Oats are also helpful for milk production if you are hoping to breastfeed.

Serves 4

1 cup [160 g] steel-cut oats
1/2 cup [90 g] chia seeds
1/2 cup [90 g] millet
1/4 cup [40 g] flax seeds
1/2 teaspoon sea salt
8 pitted Medjool dates, roughly chopped
12 Turkish apricots, roughly chopped
1/2 cup [60 g] raw whole almonds, roughly chopped

1 tart-sweet apple (like Pink Lady or Honeycrisp)
4 cups [960 ml] whole milk or milk alternative (almond or cashew milk), plus more as needed
1 tablespoon maple syrup
1 teaspoon blackstrap molasses
1/4 teaspoon vanilla extract
Fresh seasonal berries, for garnish

Combine the oats, chia seeds, millet, flax seeds, salt, dates, apricots, and almonds in a bowl. Grate the apple and add it to the porridge mixture. Pour the milk over it, then stir in the maple syrup, molasses, and vanilla. Refrigerate overnight. The next morning the grains will have swelled and may be a little thick; loosen the porridge with a little more milk. Top with the fresh berries and serve immediately. For leftover porridge, cover with enough milk to top and let it continue soaking until your next meal.

The Big Chill

In those first bleary weeks of new parenthood, a freezer full of delicious meals is a great thing to have. And there's no time like the present to start stockpiling. Here are a few ideas:

- **Soups** Soups defrost well and can be a complete meal. Try kale and white bean, Italian wedding, or classic chili.

- **Casseroles** These don't have to be 1950s tuna surprise nightmares. Vegetable-heavy lasagna or Swiss chard and sweet potatoes with eggs are both warming and nutritious.

- **Patties or meatballs** These are a great way to prepare both vegetables and meat; they are delicious and freeze well. Make your own quinoa and black bean burger or an Asian-inspired chicken meatball with chiles.

#getitdone

For clarity and a bit of direction, here are a few things to tackle this month that will help keep you organized.

Month Nine:

- Set up an autoreply for your email.
- Make and freeze some meals for postpartum.

Mama Mantra

Take what you need and let the rest go.

PART THREE

Preparing for the Birth

In my experience, many expectant mothers tend to fall into one of two camps: those who have envisioned their birth in fine detail and those who stare back at me when I ask about their birth preferences. Whether you fall into one of these or are somewhere along the spectrum between them, understanding your options and setting your intentions for your birthing experience in advance is key to feeling informed and prepared. And of course, you might find yourself worried—that's normal and I invite you to nurture yourself through the worry by allowing it to be there. No need to extinguish it, in fact embrace it—worry is here to stay. The most important thing is not to let it drive your decision-making; make choices from an informed and empowered place versus one of worry. In the following chapters, I'll help you do that by guiding you through choosing a birth team and environment, and I'll break down the key phases and concepts of labor. We'll discuss various comfort measures and techniques and, most importantly, we'll get you in the right mind-set for birth—emphasizing, as usual, the incredible power of your own intuition. Trust yourself and trust your body, and you will be well set for this great adventure.

CHAPTER SEVEN

Choose It,
Then Let It Go

———

Here is a statement that I can almost certainly guarantee is true: Your birth will not be how you imagined it.

You might imagine that giving birth in a hospital means being trapped under blue-green fluorescent lights, hooked up to imposing medical machinery. In fact, a hospital can be a soothing environment, and there are ample ways to customize your experience there, which we'll get into in the next chapter. Home births, meanwhile, may call to mind a mystical experience complete with burning aromatic incense and a wooden birthing stool and outdoor birthing tub. That's possible, but, like a hospital birth, a home birth is quite customizable and allows you to labor in the comfort of your own bed, surrounded by all of your familiar creature comforts. You may have very specific hopes for your birth—or a pile of nagging fears and preconceptions. In my experience, the best way to deal with both is to fully inform yourself of your options and establish a baseline of your own birth preferences, rooted not in firm expectations but in flexibility and curiosity.

You'll notice I use the phrase "birth preferences," not the usual "birth plan," which calls to mind a meticulously typed document outlining exactly how the mom-to-be wants to experience her birth. My choice is very intentional.

You see, I don't believe in birth plans. I believe in preferences, birth preferences that are rooted in flexibility. It's OK to have hopes for your birth, and to make informed decisions and preferences that you believe in. It can be helpful to visualize the big moment and get your thoughts and preferences on paper, but it's important to know that, as tempted as you might be to tightly embrace those preferences, you will also need to be able to completely let them go.

Pregnancy allows you to develop and exercise a new "mother muscle" as you nurture and make decisions on behalf of someone else in real time, which is something you may never have done before. What you will continue to learn over and over again as a mother is that you are not always in control. But despite that lack of control, you are going to do the best you can with the information you have. You might have a vision for how you want yourself, your life, or your baby to be. That vision may or may not become reality—particularly during childbirth, when there are so many unpredictable variables. But either way, the outcome will be yours alone—just like your baby—and as close as possible to how you've hoped it would be.

IT'S ALL NATURAL: A LOVE LETTER

When I first started training as a doula, I found myself quietly uncomfortable with the concept of "natural birth," which describes an unmedicated, vaginal birth with no medical intervention, typically performed by a midwife. During my training, it was introduced to me in the context of 1970s feminism, which was in direct contention with hospital care, or what was known as the "medical industrial complex." In that context, the central tenet of natural birthing is that women's bodies are designed for birth, and that interventions are not only unnecessary but at times traumatic. It was difficult for me to pinpoint what made me feel so unsure about it, but over the years, I've realized that the concept establishes a rigid rubric for achievement, and with that an implicit hierarchy and competitiveness for the birthing experience. As much as I loved reading about natural births—from those that happened on Ina May Gaskin's idyllic Tennessee farm to powerful yet idealistic tales in Elizabeth Davis and Debra Pascall-Bonaro's film and book *Orgasmic Birth*— and as much as I recognize the beauty, simplicity, and essential nature of it, I kept seeing women around me for whom a "natural birth" was an intensely challenging goal. If their birth experience fell short of their perceived notion of a successful birth, they had unnecessary feelings of failure and shame.

Conformity, competition, and comparison don't belong in the birthing space or dialogue. Our bodies have their own unique, innate capabilities and restrictions; therefore it seems bizarre that women should be pressured to conform to or strive for a particular kind of birthing experience. It's true that many women do successfully have unmedicated vaginal births. Our bodies are designed for it and, in the majority of cases, it is entirely possible. But what if your doctor recommends a c-section? Or what if things aren't progressing as they should and you need Pitocin, a drug that induces labor? Further, what if your birth experience would benefit from some pain management and you decide to use an epidural? I have spoken with too many women who feel a sense of failure—or worse, think that they are already "bad mothers"—because they ultimately relied on the "medical establishment," or their birth required some element of intervention. This simply isn't true— and don't let anyone tell you otherwise.

Which brings me to one of the core tenets of my doula practice: All birth is natural. It's as simple as that. Growing a baby (or multiples!) in your belly, giving a new person(s) life and bringing them into this world is an act of nature, no matter what your means of delivery: unmedicated, medicated, or cesarean birth. You have the inherent right to choose how you want to navigate your birth experience and manage or not manage your pain, and those choices should be free of judgment. You should be celebrated for moving through the process of pregnancy and birth, however you choose to do it. I encourage you to embrace this permission for yourself and to offer the same permission and empathy to our community of mothers at large. In fact, let's solidify this feeling. Read through and cosign this love letter to Natural Birth:

Dear NB,

I'm giving myself permission to have exactly the type of birth that's right for me, be it unmedicated, medicated, or a cesarean birth. Only I can choose how I want to navigate my body during my birth, and my choices are not up for comparison, shaming, or scrutiny, especially when they are beyond my control. I am capable of growing life in my body, and my body is built to birth, and that is what I believe to be natural.

Signed,

_____

[your name here]

If you feel inspired, write your own love letter to Natural Birth or your version of an ideal birth. Write it in your journal so you can revisit it throughout your pregnancy. As you write it, if you feel pressure or experience self-doubt, remember to release yourself from the ingrained tendency to strive for achievement. Allow yourself to be creative. Give yourself permission to trust your instincts, follow your internal compass, and make plans and decisions that are wholly and uniquely right for you. Becoming a mother is one of the most important moments in a woman's life. Honoring your unique birth experience, whatever it turns out to be, will help ensure that your first day of motherhood—the day you give birth to your baby—feels as empowering as it truly is.

LISTEN TO YOUR INTUITION

Deep within you and every mother I've met lies the innate ability to know and execute what's best for her and her baby. The problem is that, for most of us, reading and interpreting what I call your "internal compass" (also known as trusting your gut or listening to your inner voice) isn't something we've had a lot of practice doing. For most of our lives, we're given rules to follow, told how things are supposed to be done, and encouraged to abide by them. Even though you possess this innate ability, it can be a bit daunting to turn off the noise of outside influences and tune in to yourself. After all, advice that's dry, dogmatic, or prescriptive does simplify things. As childless adults, we can sometimes get by without regularly checking in with ourselves, but now, with your baby about to arrive, it's time to start.

For many women, pregnancy awakens a sense of strength and confidence that they haven't had before. An intuitive "gut" sheds light on different situations, places, people, and feelings in your life. Pregnant women often use a similar phrase with me: "Something tells me I need to do _____." If you haven't yet experienced this, I encourage you to try cultivating it. Pregnancy can be the beginning of a rich inner dialogue that will benefit you long after your baby is born. There are so many important decisions you will have to make during the course of your pregnancy that are based only and entirely on you, what you need, and what feels right for your body. For this reason, your intuition can be your best tool and biggest advocate during this crucial time.

Intuition is: neutral, objective, subtle.

Intuition is not: critical, shaming, fearful.

Here are a few ways you can cultivate and listen to your intuition:

Mindfulness. In Chapter Three, I introduced the concept of mindfulness—the practice of self-observation and self-awareness. If you're able, try to find time in your day to practice mindfulness techniques, like noticing your breath or mentally scanning your body for signs of tension. Mindfulness gets easier the more you do it, and once you get the hang of it, eventually it will help you slow down and reflect before reacting, even when you're in the midst of a potentially fast-paced or stressful situation.

Read, research, and reflect. In the following chapters, we'll dig into the nitty-gritty of labor and delivery—everything from the stages of labor to what to pack for your baby's first day on earth. As we unpack the details of birth, try to continually check in with yourself. Ask yourself if one option sounds more comfortable to you than another; what resonates with you, what doesn't. And a little pro tip: This is great fodder for your #writeandrelease journal, if you're keeping one.

Let a silent voice speak up. A powerful, visceral way to strengthen your relationship with your intuition is to notice your body in various situations. Confronted with a situation that triggers emotion—whether it's a place, person, or even object—pay attention to how your body reacts. Does your stomach tighten into knots? Do your shoulders tense up toward your ears? Do your lips shrink and disappear into each other? This is called body speak, and it is, quite literally, your body telling you, "Hey, I'm feeling something!"

Interview yourself. Make like a hard-nosed journalist and ask yourself the toughest questions you can think of. As an exercise, write down your questions and "ask" them of yourself days later. If your sense of conviction is starting to impress or surprise you, you're on the right track.

Ask others to interview you. If challenging yourself isn't going anywhere, that's OK. You'll get there. In the meantime, ask your doula, a trusted friend, or your partner to talk to you about birth, motherhood, and your vision for it. You might even try to seek out someone whose worldview differs from your own—you'll be surprised how quickly your sense of intuition snaps into place!

Challenging Questions to Help Hone Your Intuition

The next time you're faced with a tough decision, run through these questions:

- What makes me feel safe?

- What do I value most?

- What is the best course of action to take regarding _____?

- Is there something that I am missing or not seeing? If so, what is it?

- Do I feel stuck/confused/blocked/pressured?

- If so, can the situation be improved?

Listen Up

Was it your parents? Career counselor? Maybe even a clickbait listicle? At some point or another, we've all been encouraged to get into the habit of active listening. The motivation to actively listen is typically that you become an active participant in the conversation, and that demonstrates to the speaker that you have an interest in what they have to say. Active listening is also immensely helpful for mainlining information; that is, you will remember and internalize new information if you repeat what you hear back to yourself as you're hearing it.

Why, you may be wondering, am I lecturing you about active listening right now? When you're pregnant, you will be given lots of new information from friends, family, care providers, the Internet, and, hey, even books. Making sure that you are actively listening to new information that's being shared with you will help you fully take it in and really process it. Active listening also slows down the process of absorbing new information— after all, an internal thought happens much faster than a voiced thought. This can give you time to notice your body and feelings in reaction to this new information. Then, if you're experiencing tension, you can talk it through with a trusted family member, friend, or professional, or write what happened in your journal.

IT'S YOUR BIRTH

Throughout this book, I've encouraged you to write down your feelings. Journaling can be one of the most cathartic and fulfilling forms of therapy— and it's something you can do without spending any extra time, effort, or money. What a fantastic tool for self-support!

In the following pages, you'll find space—and I mean space in both a literal and a figurative sense—to explore, choose, and write down any and all feelings you may be experiencing related to your birth. Excitement, anxiety, obsessions—all are welcome and encouraged. You'll find nine prompts in the pages that follow and space to explore. I hope you'll find the process both grounding and illuminating.

Finally, once you've considered, reacted, and written about each of the prompts, I'll ask you to do a final step (the one mentioned in the title of this chapter): Let it go. The most positive births are experienced by women with strong convictions rooted in the utmost flexibility. Know yourself, know your limits, and be open and curious about what's to come. Release yourself from your own expectations of your birth experience.

- During this birth, what do I need from myself? What do I need from my partner? What do I need from my birth team? What do I need from my baby? What does my baby need from me?

  _____

  _____

  _____

  _____

  _____

- Start imagining the details of your ideal birth. When does it start? And where? What do you do in your early labor—watch movies? Walk in a favorite park? Rock in your baby's nursery? What brings you comfort during this time?

  _____

  _____

  _____

  _____

  _____

  _____

- What's your last meal before labor? How long will labor last, and what will your favorite part be?

  _____

  _____

  _____

  _____

  _____

  _____

- When, if applicable, do you move to your birth center or hospital? What are the intake staff like? How is your experience a positive one? Or negative? Who is with you now?

  _____

  _____

  _____

  _____

  _____

  _____

- How do you imagine your active labor? What comfort measures feel right? How do you feel emotionally during this time?

  _____

  _____

  _____

  _____

  _____

  _____

- Is your labor long? Short? Do you visualize pain? How do you imagine your reaction to it?

  _____

  _____

  _____

  _____

  _____

  _____

- What do your contractions feel like?

  _____

  _____

  _____

  _____

  _____

  _____

- In the last phase of your labor, you're pushing. What are you feeling? How do you visualize this part of your labor?

  _____

  _____

  _____

  _____

  _____

  _____

- Do you worry about complications? How do you think you'll react to them? Who is there to support you? What role do they play in more difficult moments?

_____

_____

_____

_____

_____

_____

Mama Mantra

This might be my
first time, but I know
what to do.

CHAPTER EIGHT

Choosing Your Birth Environment, Birth Team, and Preferences for You and Your Baby

In the not-too-distant past, there was one way to give birth: on your back, on a gurney, in the hospital. Before hospitals existed, birth happened at home, without any technological or medical support. These days, we're living in an exciting childbirthing era in which we have several wonderful and supportive options for not just birth environments but also members of your birth team. Read on for a detailed description of these options, and empower yourself to make educated decisions that feel right for you and your baby.

BUILDING BIRTH PREFERENCES FOR YOU AND YOUR BABY

Throughout your pregnancy, and especially as you draw closer to your due date, people from all walks of life will start to ask you about your birth plan. I don't believe in birth plans. A plan is a prescriptive, rigid outline based on a predictable outcome. Birth is nothing like that; it's unique, fluid, and unpredictable. For this reason, I like to think in terms of preferences—essential elements you'd like to implement or exclude if things go as expected (and perhaps some secondary preferences, in the case of complications). Before going into labor, it's perfectly reasonable—and, I think, important—for you to think through the realities of labor, reviewing everything we've talked about in this part of the book, and put together a general idea of what you would like for your birth and your newborn baby.

Choosing Your Birth Environment

Whether you're in a hospital room, birth center, or your bedroom, you can create an environment that resonates, uplifts, and ultimately fuels your labor. You would be surprised how seemingly trivial things like lighting and temperature can effect a laboring mother's ability to focus and work through a particularly challenging contraction. Look through this final list of possibilities and—in conjunction with some of the more clinical knowledge you now have from previous sections—try to begin visualizing your preferred birth space.

People

It's important that you feel comfortable with the people in the room while you labor. If anyone is making you feel fearful or stressed, it can slow down your labor by driving up your adrenaline, a hormone that's antagonistic to the flow of oxytocin, the hormone responsible for helping your uterus contract. If someone is making you uncomfortable, consider asking them, or having your partner or doula ask them, to give you some space. In the hospital, don't hesitate to ask for a different nurse or other personnel if need be; it's within your rights.

Lighting

Go for low: Dim lighting can help create peaceful surroundings and helps oxytocin to flow.

Temperature

Adjust the temperature as much as you need to—your body temperature will fluctuate as you labor, and it's important that you stay comfortable.

Smells

Again, a blend of lavender and clary sage can help create a supportive birthing environment; lavender helps promote relaxation, and clary sage helps promote contractions. See the Aromatherapy section (pages 280 to 281) for more information and further tips.

Sounds

Decreasing noise and stimulation can help create a more relaxing labor environment. You might consider making a playlist in advance. A mix of songs you love can really help lighten the mood.

Food and Drink

Complex carbohydrates, protein, and natural sugars are great energy providers. See Nourishment in the Comfort Menu (page 250) for specific ideas.

Preferences for Your Baby

Once your baby arrives, there are many things to consider in terms of newborn care as well, especially in your baby's first few hours of life. It's best to research and review the standard newborn care procedures at your hospital or birth center and to create a comprehensive (yet simple and quick to absorb) list of requests for how your baby is handled. Most procedures are routine, not mandatory, and if your birth goes smoothly, you should have some flexibility for if, when, and how they happen. Ideally, you want to have what many call the "golden hour," which means delaying routine newborn care procedures and prioritizing skin-to-skin bonding for up to one hour.

Here are some common concepts to be aware of in terms of newborn care.

Skin to Skin

Immediately after birth, have your baby placed on your bare chest, covered by a blanket. Research shows that skin-to-skin contact, especially in the first hour of life and particularly in the first months of life, provides incredible benefits for both mother and baby. It stabilizes a baby's breathing, temperature, and blood sugar right away, and can also contribute to accelerated brain development, lowered risk of colic, decreased overall stress, regulated body temperature, increase in the likelihood of breastfeeding, increase in milk production, and a reduced risk of postpartum depression. So basically, you should do it.

Cord Clamping

Before the umbilical cord is cut, it's clamped. An increasing body of research suggests delaying clamping and cutting the cord—until either it has stopped pulsating (three to five minutes) or the placenta has been delivered—is beneficial for your baby's health, including up to one-third greater volume of iron-rich blood from the placenta.

Cord Blood Banking

Umbilical cords are rich in stem cells, which are incredibly powerful in helping combat a wide range of maladies. As soon as you become pregnant, you'll likely start seeing online banner ads and little leaflets in your prenatal vitamins advertising some big business in stem cells: private cord blood banking. These are services that hold your baby's blood in case of emergency. They're private, so they can be used only by your family. There are also public cord blood banking options, where the cells could be used for helping other families in need or for further research in this field.

Apgar Score

This is a number given to your baby just after birth, based on an assessment of five vital signs—complexion, heart rate, reflexes, muscle tone, and respiration—which together quantify his overall health.

Weighing

After birth, your baby will be weighed on a heated scale. This doesn't take long and is typically performed in the room with you.

Bath

Your baby is born with a waxy skin covering called the vernix, a natural barrier to disease and the world's best moisturizer. It's best, if possible, to delay bathing your baby until you're well situated at home (or at the very least, no longer in the delivery room), to allow the vernix to be absorbed, and to give you and your baby time immediately after birth to bond and begin to get your breast milk flowing.

Hepatitis B Vaccine

A hepatitis B vaccination is recommended for every baby to prevent potential liver infection, cirrhosis, or liver cancer. Without getting into the vaccine debate, I will let you know that you do not have to have your baby's first hours on earth include multiple shots. Unless you, your partner, or someone else who will be close to your baby in his first week risks infecting him, he can receive this vaccine later from his pediatrician.

Vitamin K Injection

Babies are typically given a vitamin K injection after delivery. It's essential for helping blood clot (preventing hemorrhage), and very little of the vitamin passes to the infant through the placenta. Oral doses are generally available, but not preferred because they tend to be less potent.

PKU

The phenylketonuria test, generally just called a PKU, is done by pricking the newborn's heel with a small needle and collecting a blood sample. This can determine whether the baby has the necessary enzyme to convert an amino acid called phenylalanine into another amino acid, tyrosine. In individuals with phenylketonuria, phenylalanine can build up in the blood and cause brain damage, seizures, and intellectual disability. A special diet is needed to avoid these problems.

Eye Antibiotic

An antibiotic cream is applied to the newborn's eyes. While it's sometimes stated that the reason is to guard against bacteria from the rectal region, it's mainly to prevent chlamydia or gonorrhea from causing blindness. And although you likely don't have either of those (you were already screened during pregnancy), it's a public health concern and, depending on the state, may be mandatory.

Circumcision

The decision to circumcise is personal and can depend on your religious or cultural affiliation. It is not a standard procedure, although upward of 65 percent of newborn boys are circumcised. Contrary to popular belief, a circumcised penis is not cleaner than one with an intact foreskin; it really is a personal preference. The procedure itself is short and precise, typically using a specialized clamp. Circumcision has been confirmed to be painful for the baby. Numbing agents can be used if you ask for them.

Bonding

After you've decided the routine care procedures that feel right for you and your baby after birth, consider adding to your birth preferences some time to breathe, pause, and take in your baby. If all goes well, you can have immediate skin-to-skin time. Request that your birth team lower their voices, keep the lights low, and allow you at least 5 minutes of uninterrupted time to gaze into your baby's eyes and to start connecting.

YOUR BIRTH LOCATION

There's a lot to consider when selecting your birth location—your values, care needs, comfort, and, let's face it, insurance and financial parameters, especially in the United States. (Financial constraints might not be that much of a concern if you live in a country where your health care costs are heavily subsidized.) Most healthy women experiencing a complication-free pregnancy can consider any of the common birth environments: home, birth center, and hospital. If you have a medical condition, or you know in advance you'll require a c-section, or you simply feel at ease knowing that medical technology is a call-button away, a hospital is ideal. If you feel most comfortable surrounded by your own belongings and would like minimal interruption during your labor, a home birth could be right for you. And if you want something in between—less technology, with a midwife at the helm—a birth center might be a good fit.

Let's take a moment to review each environment. Reading through the details of each place, try some of your mindfulness techniques from Parts One and Two. What emotions are coming up for you, and what's really resonating (or not) as you read through the realities of the different settings?

The Hospital

In this environment, care is typically physician-led, with nurses implementing the physician's orders. Depending on your location, there may be a midwife on staff to assist and manage your birth.

The Ins and Outs of Birthing at a Hospital

- Your care is provided by a board-certified doctor (OB/GYN) and a team of labor and delivery nurses.

- You may also have a doula or supportive labor partner present.

- Hospitals are equipped to diagnose and treat you and your baby if serious complications occur. For example, if surgery is needed for you or your baby you'll have access to an operating room.

- There's no need to transfer to another facility before, during, or after labor.

- You'll have direct access to pain medications that are not available in nonhospital settings (such as epidurals).

- Hospital care includes many safety protocols—some that require more intervention than others. The use of IV fluids, Pitocin, or breaking the amniotic sac (commonly called the "bag of waters") may be encouraged or advised for you.

- Various levels of technology (fetal monitoring, blood pressure, and so on) are integrated into care and, depending on your care provider, can drive labor decisions over your body's physiology or your instincts—for example, if you'd prefer to change positions, but an IV or monitoring device prevents this from happening. In these instances, doula support is especially helpful in navigating medical decision-making that works for you and for your health needs.

- Your access to food or drink might be limited.

- You may spend time in a small triage room having blood drawn or vitals checked before moving to your actual delivery room.

- The nursing support staff will be caring for other patients and therefore may not be continually available for your support.

- Your hospital room may not be that spacious, and you may be in it for a long time.

- You will travel to the hospital while your labor is under way and return home after birth.

Get Friendly with Your Baby

If you are choosing to breastfeed, take a look at Baby Friendly, USA, a subsidiary of the World Health Organization's Baby Friendly Health Initiative. BFUSA is an accrediting body that works with hundreds of hospitals in the United States to determine if they are following proper guidelines that support breastfeeding mothers and newborns. To be a baby-friendly hospital (BFH), the hospital must have some element of lactation or breastfeeding support and typically encourages practices like skin-to-skin mother-baby contact right after birth, rooming in, and other practices that help jump-start a great breastfeeding practice. To find hospitals in your area that work with BFUSA's guidelines, visit babyfriendlyusa.org.

What to Pack for a Hospital Birth

For Labor	After Delivery	For Baby and the Return Home
Snacks and drinks (coconut water, bananas, bars, fruit)	Nightgown/PJs (with easy chest access)	Footed, kimono-style onesies (2)
Lip balm	Robe	Hats (2)
Socks with traction grip	Nursing bra and nursing pads	Socks (2)
Hair bands	Nipple cream, breast shells if needed	Mittens (2)
Birth ball	Nursing pillow	6 to 10 diapers (if you have a brand preference, otherwise the hospital will provide)
Camera (if you have one you love more than the camera on your phone)	Towel (hospital towels tend to be thin; a cozy towel from home might make you feel at ease)	Receiving/swaddling blankets (2)

For Labor	After Delivery	For Baby and the Return Home
Aromatherapy diffuser and chosen essential oils and massage oils	Toilet paper (they usually have one-ply, so if you want something softer, bring it)	Car seat (preinstalled)
Electric candles (soften the ambience)	Personal toiletries (face wash, lotion, moisturizer, makeup basics)	Your ID and insurance card
Disposable underwear	Going home outfit	Baby carrier (soft wrap, great for partners if you have an extended stay)

Remember, You're Healthy!

At the hospital, it can be very easy to think of yourself as sick or unwell. It makes sense because we associate hospitals with sickness. But, you're not sick—although the hospital is for illness. You are well and your hospital birth team is to there to help you have your baby.

The Birth Center

A birth center is a midwife-led facility featuring a cozy, home-like environment (in fact, many are located in converted homes) and some degree of medical capability. Many hospitals have a birth center inside their facility that is operated by midwives, which can be an ideal option for someone seeking a blend of a home birth and hospital birth experience. (Be advised that some of these facilities are "birth centers" in name only and are actually just a normal hospital delivery unit; in that case, there may be differences from the list that follows. Don't be afraid to ask questions and make sure you know what is truly on offer.)

The Ins and Outs of Birthing at a Birth Center

- Your care is provided by licensed midwives.

- You may also have a doula or supportive labor partner present.

- Your care is administered based on your expressed preferences.

- Technology is used sparingly; focus is placed on your intuition and your body's physiology.

- Interventions like Pitocin or epidurals are unavailable; alternative methods of pain management—such as nitrous oxide, movement, massage, and hydrotherapy—are encouraged.

- Your birth team, which typically comprises your midwife and doula, is available to give you continuous physical, emotional, and informational support during your labor and birth, and to support your companions as well.

- Time is less of a consideration; you're encouraged to labor for as long as is needed if you and your baby are coping well.

- You'll be able to eat and drink as you please.

- If there are any complications during or after labor, you will be transferred to a hospital. Sometimes your midwife's chosen hospital may not have the personnel available to provide immediate care.

- Freestanding birth centers do not have access to emergency care facilities like an operating room, neonatal intensive care unit (NICU), or pediatric support.

- You will travel to the birth center as your labor begins and return home after birth.

What to Pack for the Birth Center

For Labor	After Delivery	For Baby and the Return Home
Snacks and drinks (coconut water, bananas, bars, fruit)	Nightgown/PJs (with easy chest access)	Footed, kimono-style onesies (2)
Lip balm	Robe	Hats (2)
Socks with traction grip	Nursing bra and nursing pads	Socks (2)
Hair bands	Nipple cream and breast shells if needed	Mittens (2)
Birth ball	Nursing pillow	6 to 10 diapers (if you have a brand preference, otherwise the birth center will provide)
Camera	Towel	Receiving/swaddling blankets (2)
Aromatherapy diffuser and chosen essential oils, and massage oils	First meal (made and frozen ahead—protein-rich soups are perfect)	Car seat (preinstalled)
Electric candles	Personal toiletries	Your ID and insurance card
Disposable underwear	Going home outfit	Baby carrier

Note: *Consider packing a second, lighter bag with a few essentials, should you need to transfer to a hospital quickly.*

At Home

Birthing at home is similar to birthing at a birth center, but you're in your own intimate and familiar space. This type of birth requires a deep energetic commitment from you, your partner, and anyone else you would like present at your birth. Everyone needs to feel confident and united in your decision. If this isn't the case, it can create an unsafe emotional environment, which can make your labor more challenging than it needs to be. Why? Because key labor hormones like oxytocin don't function optimally when you feel physically or emotionally unsafe; instead, your body releases more fight-or-flight hormones like cortisol, which can slow and even stall your labor. A steadfast alliance makes all the difference, and should you unite on this decision, an at-home environment can provide you with a sense of ease and allow you to create a unique and unrestricted space for your birth.

The Ins and Outs of Birthing at Home

- Your care is provided by licensed midwives or certified nurse midwives.

- You may also have a doula or supportive labor partner present.

- You have the comforts of your own home at your disposal, such as your bathtub/shower and your own bed, which can bring solace during a longer labor.

- Your birth is looked at individually, and your midwife tailors the care to your expressed preferences and needs.

- Focus is placed on your intuition and your body's physiology.

- The use of interventions is avoided, and in most cases they are not made available.

- You'll be able to eat and drink as you please.

- Your birth team, which typically comprises your midwife and doula, are available to give you continuous physical, emotional, and informational support during your labor and birth, and to support your companions as well.

- Time is less of a consideration; you're encouraged to labor for as long as is needed if you and baby are coping well.

- The entirety of your labor, birthing, and recovery takes place in your home.

- If there are any complications during or after labor, you will have to transfer to a hospital. Sometimes your midwife's chosen hospital may not have the personnel available to provide immediate care.

- Solidifying a support team with your midwife, a transfer hospital, and a physician might be complicated, particularly if your midwife works closely with only a single provider and that person is unavailable during your birth.

- You won't have any access to pain medications nor immediate access to emergency care facilities.

- The proximity of your home to the hospital might not be ideal, in case of complications.

- You may have to purchase a fairly extensive list of preparatory items, like a birthing tub and a premade birthing kit, which your midwife will require and direct you to purchase.

- You will have to prepare a secondary hospital bag, in case you need to be transferred to the hospital.

What to Have Available for a Home Birth

For Labor	After Delivery	Secondary Hospital Bag and Other Necessities for an Emergency
Birth tub and liner	First meal (made and frozen ahead—protein-rich soups are perfect)	Toiletries
Hose to fill tub	Nursing bra and nursing pads	Your ID and insurance card
Plastic sheets	Nipple cream and breast shells if needed	Car seat (preinstalled)
Aromatherapy and massage oils	1 set of sheets for after birth	6 to 10 diapers (if you have a brand preference, otherwise the hospital will provide)
Plastic mattress cover or thick polyethylene firm mattress	1 set of pillowcases for after birth	Going home outfit for you and baby
4 to 6 adult-size bath towels	Disposable underwear	Receiving/swaddling blankets
4 to 6 washcloths	Receiving/swaddling blankets (2)	Nightgown/PJs (with easy chest access)

#writeandrelease

- When I've received care in the past, what did I enjoy the most and the least?

- What do I (and possibly my partner) need to feel comfortable in a care setting?

The Many Faces of Midwifery

You may already be familiar with the concept of a midwife—a person trained to provide medical, mental, cultural, emotional, and even spiritual needs during pregnancy and delivery. What you may not know is that there are many different educational requirements and board exams that enable someone to be a midwife—and there are many derivations. Here's a brief primer.

A **Certified Midwife** has been certified by the American Midwifery Certification Board, and provides birth support in a hospital setting.

A **Certified Nurse-Midwife (CNM)** is an advanced-practice certified nurse who specializes in midwifery. Essentially these are certified, registered nurses who have also passed the American Midwifery Certification Board exams. A CNM provides birth support in a hospital setting or a freestanding birth center.

A **Certified Professional Midwife (CPM)** is an independent practitioner. A CPM meets the accreditation requirements of the North American Registry of Midwives. This is the only midwifery accreditation that requires both knowledge and practice in nonhospital settings.

Licensed midwives and **registered midwives** are both a type of direct-entry midwife. They are independent practitioners who have trained themselves through self-study in the Midwife Model of Care, and they primarily—almost exclusively—work outside of hospitals.

Finally, **traditional midwives** are those who have no accreditation, but are trained through support of the community and their cultural context.

THE BIRTH TEAM

Choosing the members of your birth team feels a lot like dating. And, at the beginning, there's a good amount of swiping left and Google stalking as you narrow your field. Luckily for you, I've got a method that's better than trolling Yelp (although feel free to incorporate that site into your process as well): the four Rs—Resources, Reputation, Resonance, Referrals. Makes it seem fairly easy, right? It should definitely help.

Resources

As in: yours. If you're in the U.S., what type of insurance do you have, and what does it cover? What hospitals or birth centers are available to you, and what care providers? It's not very glamorous and doesn't require much soul-searching or intuition-honing, but it's truly where you should start, and I encourage you to get this part squared away before moving on to more personal decisions. Some women choose to pay out of pocket for care, as some notable care providers don't accept insurance. It's important that you get a realistic idea of what your means are for your birth so that you can choose the most appropriate option from within that pool.

Reputation

I like to start with my own network when searching for care providers. If you're comfortable, I would even go so far as to ask your friends via Facebook: Update your status and ask around. Seriously! Nowhere else will you find a tailor-made group of people ready to answer within the hour who also know you, your background, and maybe even your preferences. Once you've got some ideas, you can cross-reference ratings and reviews online. Yes, even on Yelp. Take a look at Vitals, which aggregates scores from other medical review sites. One caveat for such online forums: Medical advice is not a restaurant review, and we all know the shortcomings of public review sites. Be savvy, take it with a grain of salt, and ultimately, listen to your intuition.

Resonance

You've found a care provider you think you're on board with. Great! Now it's time to have a meeting. Most care providers are happy to do it, although some of the very busy or notable OBs don't take interviews. Now, of course, this person isn't joining your family; you aren't going to be dating them long term. But they'll play an important role in the next year of your life, so it's important that you see eye to eye; you're looking for a connection. You can even take it step by step. How do you feel in the lobby, in the exam room, in their office? Do you cut tension with levity? Do they?

Referrals

No matter whom you choose to work with—doctor, midwife, doula—you are hoping for them to be your referral base for further care. You may need to see a specialist, see someone for genetic testing, or visit a chiropractor or acupuncturist. You will want to make sure that the care provider you choose resonates with you to the extent that you also trust their opinion of other providers in their network.

Commitment Issues

It's important to note that you can switch providers at (almost) any time. Up to thirty-seven gestational weeks, in fact. You are not stuck. Just knowing this can seriously take the edge off of deciding on a birth team member.

Doctor

No matter how you may feel about the health care system, there is an intrinsic power dynamic between a doctor and a patient. Their knowledge—you know, the reason you sought them out—can be intimidating for some people and can make them feel powerless. As a pregnant person, it's not unusual to feel vulnerable in your doctor's office, to feel like you can't really speak your mind. For this reason and even more generally, I believe that the most important element of choosing your doctor is communication. The hope is that you can choose a health care provider who creates a supportive space where you can feel able to communicate—to speak your mind, approach hesitations and fears, and ultimately, communicate freely with your doctor in a way that feels right for you. Additionally, you may want to evaluate the doctor's overall communication style. She may be brisk in her exam with you, yet available any time via text. Or he may have lengthy and supportive appointments with you, yet not be reachable after office hours except for in emergencies or labor.

Lastly, the primary perspective of your doctor will be focused on the goal of a healthy, thriving mother and a healthy, thriving baby. Clearly, those are important priorities. However, if you're looking for a more dynamic experience, it can be fun to seek out a doctor who has other interests or dual specialties, depending on what's important for you, such as an interest in naturopathy, fitness, or clean eating.

A Few Great Questions for Your Doctor

Her Philosophy

- What is your general philosophy about pregnancy and birth?

- What is your elective induction rate? Emergency c-section rate? How do you feel about both?

- Do you support unmedicated birth if that's what our goal is?

- How do you feel about epidurals? What kind are available at your hospital?

- How many years have you been practicing?

- Are you a parent? How old are your children now? How were they born?

- Do you work alone or with a partner or assistant? What is their experience? Will you be at my birth, or does it depend on who's on call?

- What is your experience with breech births?

- How many patients/clients do you have now? Do you have a maximum, and how do you manage to avoid too many commitments?

- How often will I see you? What do your checkups consist of? How much time do I have with you? Is it OK to ask questions?

- Do you suggest that I take a childbirth education class? Do you teach such a class?

- Who takes over for you if you go on vacation or get sick?

Your Care

- Do you support me going to forty-two weeks if the baby and I are doing well?

- As long as my baby and I are doing well, how much freedom do I have during labor? (Eating, moving around, tub, and so on.)

>>>

- How do you feel about doulas?

- When should I call you after my labor begins? When should I come to the hospital?

- Are you patient with labor to let it progress on its own time, as long as my baby and I are doing well?

- What are your thoughts on cord clamping and cord blood banking?

- How much time do you allow for the delivery of the placenta?

- What are my options if my water breaks?

- What would you consider a good reason to induce?

- If I am Strep B positive, what effect will that have on my baby's birth?

- What are your feelings on episiotomies?

Midwife

Midwife care differs most dramatically from obstetric care in that your midwife will be party to every aspect of your pregnancy. Again, this is something that comes down to personal preference—one is in no way better than another. A midwife will monitor everything from what you're eating and how you're sleeping to stress and how your relationship is going, as those things can all relate to and affect your pregnancy. The right OB/GYN will do this, too.

You will want to find out the logistical parameters to her care: what birth centers she works with, if she works with other midwives or student-midwives. You will also want to know what OB/GYN she works with and what hospital they're associated with, in case of emergency.

Finally, as with your doctor, you will want to know about her level of communication. Is she readily available to answer your (at times panicked, at times off-hours) questions? Don't assume a specific level of care simply because she is a midwife and not a doctor.

A Few Great Questions for Your Midwife

Her Philosophy

- What is your general philosophy about pregnancy and birth?

- How many years have you been practicing?

- Are you a parent? How old are your children now? How were they born?

- Do you work alone or with a partner or assistant? What is their experience? Will you be at my birth, or does it depend on who's on call?

- What is your experience with breech births?

- How many patients/clients do you have now? Do you have a maximum, and how do you manage to avoid too many commitments?

- How often will I see you? What do your checkups consist of? How much time do I have with you? Is it OK to ask questions?

- Do you suggest that I take a childbirth education class? Do you teach such a class?

- Who takes over for you if you go on vacation or get sick?

Your Care

- Do you support me going to forty-two weeks if the baby and I are doing well?

- As long as my baby and I are doing well, how much freedom do I have during labor? (Eating, moving around, tub, and so on.)

- How do you feel about doulas?

- When should I call you after my labor begins?

- Are you patient with labor to let it progress on its own time, as long as my baby and I are doing well?

- What are your thoughts on cord clamping and cord blood banking?

>>>

- Will you allow my partner to be as active at the birth as s/he desires?

- How much time do you allow for the delivery of the placenta?

- If I am Strep B positive, what effect will that have on my baby's birth?

Doula

A birth doula's role is very different from that of your midwife or doctor. She will provide you with nonmedical labor support, so of all of your central birth team members, she is the one for whom you'll have to really consider what support you are looking for before you find out her services. Not every doula provides the same offerings; some offer childbirth education, labor support, massage sessions, and even placenta encapsulation (turning your placenta into capsules for you to ingest) in their packages. You may or may not need all of what they offer. It's important to decide what you need from your doula. At a minimum you should have two prenatal sessions with your doula to build rapport—these don't have to be a private childbirth education class, they can be more emotionally focused—plus day-of-labor support and one follow-up visit.

Also, you may have the preconception that having a doula means birthing at home or a birth center; that's not the case at all. In my doula practice I would say about 70 percent of clients birth in the hospital; in fact, I think the hospital is where a doula can be the most helpful. Why? Because your doula is with you the entire time you're laboring; as the nursing staff changes, your doula will be your constant guide, looking out for your comfort and interests. This can be a wonderful thing, especially as most OB/GYNs will pop in and out briefly during your labor, spending more time with you only once you're ready to push.

This doesn't mean doulas aren't helpful at home or a birth center. Far from it. Remember, in labor, although the midwife model of care is more holistic and focused on the overall well-being and comfort of the laboring woman, the midwife is also focused on medical components of your birth: blood pressure and other vitals. Your doula will really be the one helping you with your breathing, movement, and massage—helping you to keep calm and centered, and making sure you stay hydrated and fed.

And again, as with all of your care providers, get a sense of your doula candidates' availability and how that relates to what they charge. Are they strict about how many in-person or phone appointments are included in their package? Will they offer postpartum support? It's important to get a strong sense of how they run their business and how you can fit in (or not).

Finally, find out who they use as their backup. Most doulas are on call (it's part of the job), but if they are ill or truly cannot attend your birth, who can you expect to offer you support in their place? It's a good idea to meet with that person before your birth as well.

A Few Great Questions for Your Doula

- Why did you become a doula?
- What sort of training have you had?
- How many births have you attended?
- Do you generally work with home births or hospital births?
- Which hospitals are you most comfortable with? Why?
- Are you part of a collective? Who is your backup?
- How many clients do you take per month?
- How much do you charge?
- What does that include?
- What kind of specialized services do you offer?
- Do you have experience in complicated births like mine? (If applicable)

>>>

- Are you supportive of medicated and unmedicated birth? If not, why?

- Will you support me through any decision?

Pediatrician

I'm a one-step-at-a-time kind of girl, so I understand if you're not ready to take on this decision now. But while you're getting referrals, going on interviews, and constructing your dream birth team, it's also a great time to look into a pediatrician. After all, this is a very important relationship (one that has the potential to last eighteen or more years!), so you might as well start looking for The One now. You need to have selected a pediatrician before your baby can come home with you, and a pediatrician will be present in the birth room during delivery and/or visit you in the hospital (and at that point, if you haven't selected one, it will be one who is assigned to you).

A Few Great Questions for Your Pediatrician

- What are the office hours? What is the contact protocol after hours?

- Who is on call after hours: a doctor or nurse?

- What hospital is the office or doctor associated with?

- What is their policy and/or philosophy on various drugs, including vaccines and antibiotics?

- What is your impression of the office staff?

- Ask questions that can give you a sense of the doctor's overall philosophy, such as "How big a deal is it if I'm unable to continue breastfeeding?" or "Is letting the baby cry it out the best sleep training method?"

Other Potential Teammates

The deeper you get into motherhood, the more you will come to believe that old saying: It takes a village. Here is a brief schematic of some care providers who may be helpful to you over the course of your pregnancy and shortly after you have your baby.

Team Member	When	What They Help With
Acupuncturist	First, second, and third trimesters	Stress and anxiety reduction, nausea in first trimester
Chiropractor	Third trimester	Low back pain and pelvic pressure
Massage therapist	Third trimester	Pain relief and anxiety reduction
Psychotherapist or pregnancy/parenting coach	Second trimester	Discuss upcoming change
Kinesiologist	Second trimester	Complementary to chiropractic
Physical therapist	Second trimester	Pelvic floor specialist
Homeopath	Second trimester	Natural relief for nausea, reflux, headache, and more

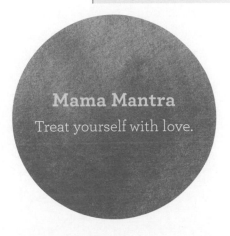

Mama Mantra
Treat yourself with love.

CHAPTER NINE

Labor:

The Signs, Stages, and Interventions

———

For many expectant mothers, the chapter that follows contains the information they're most curious about. You may even have flipped directly to this chapter when you first picked up this book. If so, you're not alone. Many first-time pregnant women are curious about the unpredictable, often unimaginable event that is labor. From the moment you found out you were pregnant, you might even have thought, "I'm going to have to do what? From where?!" Yes, you are. And you'll do great.

In the following pages, I present a clear breakdown of what women commonly experience during labor. I've laid it out simply, so that you and your partner, doula, or whomever you enlist for labor support can reference it quickly, even in the heat of the moment. You'll get an idea of your body's labor signs as you approach your due date and the three major stages of labor. If you're having a scheduled cesarean birth (or if you want to get acquainted with what happens if you end up having one unexpectedly), you'll find a section about it at the end of this chapter.

And if you did, in fact, open the book and flip directly to this page and are already feeling overwhelmed, that's also entirely OK (and normal). Head back to Chapter One and I'll meet you there. We'll get to all this later.

Know Your Lingo

Get out your flash cards; this list includes some key labor-related terminology.

Uterus is the reproductive organ in which a baby is nurtured from implantation through gestation. In birth, it works in muscular contractions to push your baby out through your vagina.

Placenta is a temporary organ. It functions as a connection between you and your baby during your pregnancy, transferring oxygen and carbon dioxide, as well as bringing in nutrients and carrying out waste. After delivery, the placenta is expelled, and any hormones that were produced by the placenta fade from your bloodstream.

Cervix is the cylindrical neck of tissue that connects the vagina and the uterus. In pregnancy, it is tightly closed, with the help of the mucus plug. In birth, it softens (effaces) and opens (dilates) to the vagina to make way for your baby's head.

The **mucus plug** is a literal plug of mucus that forms early in pregnancy to seal the opening of the cervix until labor begins.

Dilation (in centimeters) refers to the width of the cervical opening. It is determined by your doctor, midwife, or nurse manually by a vaginal exam. Your cervix will dilate from 0 (closed) to 10 (completely dilated) centimeters during labor. In first labors, the cervix dilates at an average of 1 centimeter per hour; this rate is often faster for subsequent labors.

Effacement describes the thickness, softness, and depth of the cervix, as it opens to the birth canal to accommodate your baby's head. Cervix effacement is measured on a percentile from 0 (very thick) to 100 (completely thinned out).

Pelvic station describes the vertical position of your baby's head in relation to your pelvis. This is recorded as a number between −5 and +5. Zero station means the head is "engaged" and has entered the vaginal canal within the pelvic bones. A negative number (−5 to 0) means that the head isn't engaged in the pelvis. A positive number (0 to +4) means that

>>>

your baby's head is moving down the pelvis; +5 means your baby's head is crowning (becoming visible as it emerges through the cervix, without slipping back. Ideally, you should not push until the head is engaged in the pelvis, even if you're fully dilated.

Early labor, also called latent labor, is the first period of labor, the longest and the least intense. During this stage, your cervix will dilate from 0 to 6 centimeters.

Active labor is, just as the term indicates, an active portion of the labor process when you'll experience regular, strong contractions as your cervix dilates from 7 to 10 centimeters.

THE SIGNS

How many movies or television shows have you watched that featured a scene like this? A pregnant woman who is shopping at the supermarket reaches for some item, and all of a sudden her water breaks, producing a huge gush. Jokes about "cleanup on aisle seven" follow, then a heart attack–inducing scene as she is frantically driven to the hospital.

In reality, only 7 to 10 percent of women's labors begin with the spontaneous breaking of their water—that is, the amniotic sac rupturing and releasing all its fluid. Your labor will more likely begin with a confluence of very subtle, less cinematic signs, beginning about a month out from your due date. As you approach the day, you will pass through a series of moderate signs and finally arrive at definite signs, of which water breaking is just one. The charts that follow break down each of these stages: Subtle Signs, Moderate Signs, and Positive Signs.

Subtle Signs

The Sign	What's Happening?	Tips and Comfort Measures
Restless backache	Your growing uterus is putting pressure on your low back.	Find comfort when lying down by arranging pregnancy pillows (or carefully arranged normal pillows) under your belly and between your knees.
Soft bowel movements	Your body is releasing hormone-like substances called prostaglandins, which thin the cervix in preparation for labor and can prompt activity in your bowels.	Revisit comfort measures from your first trimester (such as the ginger tea on page 85) to help fight those flu-like symptoms.
Cramps	Prostaglandins are causing trouble again, and possibly early contractions, too.	As with menstrual cramps, movement can really help. Walking, stretching, and using a birth ball are all good ideas. Hot showers help, too.
Nesting	Your body's urge to prepare for birth prompts a nesting instinct.	If you're up for it, by all means reorganize your entire house. Remember not to lift anything too heavy, and really try to get some rest, too.
Mood swings	Surging levels of oxytocin can bring irritability and crabbiness to the forefront.	Fall back on your mindfulness practice. Deep breaths and taking a moment to collect yourself can really help.
Sharp groin pain	Your baby drops lower, settling deep into your pelvis as she prepares for birth. This is called lightening.	Acid reflux and shortness of breath may be less of a problem as your lungs and stomach gain a little extra room.

Moderate Signs

Labor hasn't started, but it might be not too far out—a matter of a few weeks, days, or maybe just hours.

The Sign	What's Happening?	You May Notice	Tips and Comfort Measures
Mucus plug is discharged	Your cervix has effaced to a point where it no longer holds the "plug" that seals the opening of your uterus, which causes the plug to slip out. Some women lose their mucus plug and labor begins that day; for others, labor will begin only days or weeks later. That's why it's a moderate sign; it means your cervix is starting to change, which is great.	A blood-tinged mucus discharge released from your vagina.	The discharge of the mucus plug is often mistaken for "bloody show" (see Definite Signs). The mucus plug is a brown/beige color, whereas bloody show is pink or red.
Nonprogressing contractions, known as Braxton Hicks contractions	Your uterus is practicing for its big moment.	A tightening of the uterus that happens intermittently and irregularly, not becoming longer, stronger, or closer together over time as the contractions of labor do.	While not typically painful, Braxton Hicks contractions can be tiring, discouraging, and sometimes frightening, as they can make you think labor is under way. Although they aren't labor

The Sign	What's Happening?	You May Notice	Tips and Comfort Measures
			contractions, they still play an important prelabor role for your uterus. Typically, if you get up and walk around, the feeling will subside, which is a true indication that these are not, in fact, labor contractions.
Amniotic sac tears	This is a moderate sign because if your water breaks without progressive contractions, things are happening, but your labor has yet to begin.	A small trickle of fluid.	A maxi pad or adult diaper can help, if the leakage becomes annoying or inhibits activity.
Amniotic sac breaks	Your baby's head, as he makes his way into the pelvis, creates pressure that will cause the amniotic membrane to rupture or break. It is very rare (1 in 10) for your amniotic sac to break before labor begins.	A large gush of fluid.	Your doctor will collect some fluid from your vagina to test for amniotic fluid.

Water, Water . . . Everywhere?

Well, not really. In fact, few women experience that Hollywood moment when their amniotic sac ruptures.

If your water has broken, you might feel the following sensations:

- A trickle of clear liquid, as if you can't stop urinating.

- Increased pelvic pressure.

- Contractions that increase severely in intensity, either immediately or within a few hours.

Your water broke—you should:

- Note the time it happened.

- Discern how much fluid was lost; is it a trickle or a gush?

- Note the color and the odor: Amniotic fluid is colorless and odorless.

- Avoid having sex.

- Update your care provider and labor support team.

- Consult your care provider or visit the hospital or birth center immediately if:

  ✳ The liquid has any color or odor—it should be clear and have no smell.

  ✳ Your amniotic sac bursts without any contractions or other signs of active labor.

Depending on your care provider, you might have various plans about what to do once your water breaks; it all depends on the state of your pregnancy and your baby's health. Some doctors might want you to come to the hospital immediately. Or your midwife or doctor might say it's OK to wait a few hours for contractions to begin on their own, which can sometimes happen more easily in your home environment. This is something you can discuss with your care provider prenatally. The likelihood is that your contractions will start on their own within twelve to twenty-four hours after your water breaks.

Positive Signs

The Sign	What's Happening?	You'll Notice	Tips and Comfort Measures
Progressing contractions	Your uterus is periodically tightening, creating contractions that become longer, stronger, and closer together over time. These contractions cause the cervix to dilate and thin in preparation for birth.	Intense cramping, possibly in your low back (think menstrual cramps), quickly followed by your abdomen tightening gradually as the contraction builds.	Make the most of the rest periods between contractions. Breathe silently, lie down, or ask for a massage or aromatherapy.
Bloody show	Blood vessels in the cervix rupture as the cervix begins to dilate and efface.	A blood-tinged discharge.	This won't be painful, but can be messy or uncomfortable. A maxi pad will help you keep clean. Remember, a little bit of bloody discharge is a good sign; it means your cervix is starting to change and open.

THE STAGES

As someone who encounters birth and its processes on a daily basis, I always find it surprising how little most of the women I work with know about how it works. They know you have to be dilated, but they don't know what that means. They know there are contractions and pushing, but they may think those are two separate moments. So here is a step-by-step breakdown of the three stages of labor and how it all works, plus some feelings you may experience along the way.

The Stages of Labor

- **First stage:** cervical dilation and early and active labor

- **Second stage:** pushing and delivering your baby

- **Third stage:** delivery of the placenta

Peaks and Valleys: Visualizing Contractions

You may feel like more of a sprinter than a marathon runner, but luckily for you, your body is already an expert in endurance. When you start labor, you won't be contracting the entire time. Your body gives you breaks to recharge, collect yourself, and get ready for the next one. Think of each contraction as a mountain: As you climb, it builds in intensity, eventually peaking and then subsiding as you come down the other side. When climbing to the peak, you give all your energy—more than you may have ever done before in your life—but on the other side, in the valley, you stretch out, relax, smell the wildflowers. As you rest, you're able to reap all the benefits of your body's natural pharmacy. If you've ever done a particularly hard workout, you know that right afterward there is a rush of endorphins to boost you up. In fact, endorphins are a natural form of morphine created by your body. The valley after a contraction peak works the same way. If you're able to breathe and relax between contractions, you'll be able to reap the effect of the endorphins release, which can minimize pain and even give you a sense of euphoria.

Early Labor (First Stage)

Most likely the longest portion of your labor, the early labor period can last anywhere from several hours to several days. Contractions are quite far apart at this time and are relatively mild, resembling menstrual cramps or a low backache.

How Dilated Am I?

Cervical dilation during labor is determined by a digital vaginal examination from your doctor or midwife. While it can provide information about how far you have progressed in labor, it cannot accurately predict the length of your labor. Other factors, such as the strength, duration, and length of contractions and your overall behavior, can be a better indicator. Cervical dilation is just one way your doctor or midwife can help keep track. Frequent exams are not recommended, due to increased infection risks each time anything is inserted into your vagina (especially if your water has broken) and the discomfort of the process. You have the right to waive an exam should you not feel comfortable for any reason, if the reason for the check isn't due to an emergency. Vaginal exams can also be uncomfortable, so before you have one, you might want your partner, doula, or support person to hold your hand and breathe with you as it happens.

Early labor is characterized by:

- Contractions lasting approximately thirty to forty-five seconds

- Contractions that are approximately five to twenty minutes apart

- Cervix dilating from 0 to 6 centimeters

- Cervix beginning to soften and efface

Contractions feel like: Menstrual-like cramps or upset stomach.

Common feelings and sensations: Backache (constant or with each contraction), diarrhea, indigestion, vomiting—the stomach clearing its contents to make room for the uterus to work at its best.

Comfort measures: If you have the energy, engage in nonstressful activities that provide distraction: Cook some extra freezable meals for your first weeks of parenthood, email friends, fold baby clothes, watch TV. If you feel up for it, get out for a walk, meet a friend for lunch, or see a movie. Whatever you do, just don't push it, and always make sure your cell phone is handy.

A note for your partner: Because pain is more easily managed in this stage, the laboring mother may be able to enjoy activities like reading, watching TV, or just having a conversation or a nap—all of which can be helpful distractions.

Active Labor (First Stage)

Active labor is more akin to the intense, dramatic event you may have been imagining throughout your pregnancy. It comes with more intense contractions, which will continue to grow stronger, longer, and closer together until you feel the urge to push. This part of your labor is hard to predict, so it's best to buckle in and allow it to unfold naturally. Active labor can last anywhere from one to over eight hours, sometimes more.

Active labor is characterized by:

- Contractions lasting approximately sixty to ninety seconds, which can be irregular at first

- Contractions that are approximately three to five minutes apart

- Contractions do not go away when you lie down and increase in intensity when you walk or move

- Dilation from 6 to 10 centimeters

- Complete cervical effacement

Contractions feel like: Strong tightening in your abdomen, like you're doing a high-intensity ab crunch, or like a towel wrapped around your belly is being firmly tightened.

Common feelings and sensations: Increasing pain and discomfort, heaviness in your legs, fatigue, burping, not being able to talk during a contraction.

Comfort measures: Breathwork and movement can help you work through contractions; massage and relaxed meditation can help you unwind during rest periods. See Chapter Ten (page 234) for a range of exercises and suggestions for both medicated and unmedicated births.

A note for your partner: Time to practice your soothing encouragement techniques. During contractions, a laboring mother will likely want to hear positive reinforcement. Tell her how impressed you are by her strength, and remind her that every contraction brings her closer to meeting her baby.

When to Go to the Hospital or Birthing Center: False Labor and the Clock

The general rule of thumb is to move to your birth location when your contractions are at 5-1-1, which means they are 5 minutes apart and 1 minute long, and this has been the case for at least 1 hour. Before you reach that point, it's generally advisable—and most comfortable—for you to labor at home.

There are a handful of situations that override the 5-1-1 rule:

- Your amniotic sac breaks spontaneously. Keep in mind you still might not have to head to the hospital before contractions begin, but you should let your care provider know immediately; they can inform you about what to do next.

- You feel sharp, stabbing pain with your contractions.

- Intense rectal pressure, like you're trying to have a bowel movement, but when you do nothing comes out; this could mean that your baby's head is quite low in the birth canal and it's best to get to your birthing environment or call your midwife if you're birthing at home.

- You notice very heavy vaginal bleeding or green fluid.

- You are experiencing blurred vision, headaches, and dizziness.

>>>

It might be false labor if contractions . . .

- Are irregular and short—lasting less than forty-five seconds and happening every thirty minutes over a few hours

- Are not becoming longer, stronger, and closer together

- Go away completely when you change activity, walk around, lie down, or eat

- Create tightening in the groin or upper part of your uterus

The Clock

If you go to your birth environment too early—whether it's a birth center or hospital—you may end up being sent home. Alternatively, you may be admitted too early and, if you're giving birth at a hospital, you'll begin to encounter "the clock." The clock is active labor management; as soon as you're admitted to the hospital, the imperative is that your labor progresses in an efficient amount of time. If you arrive in early labor and there isn't measurable progress (dilation and effacement and more frequent contractions) within the first four to six hours, you may be offered interventions to help move your labor along. Therefore, laboring at home until you're in an active labor pattern (5-1-1) is ideal in order to reduce the likelihood of interventions and allow your body to do its work on its own. This is something to discuss with your care provider prenatally. If you are sent home, start using the movement circuit (see page 258), which will help move things along.

Pushing and Delivery (Second Stage)

Everyone is different, but for some women pushing can be the most rewarding part of labor, as the woman's own strong and definitive actions become the driving force birthing her baby. Some women even become more alert or talkative. You'll begin pushing only when you are completely dilated, which is determined by your care provider. Upon complete dilation, you might have a brief resting phase of ten to thirty minutes—longer if you have an epidural—when your contractions may slow down and space out. If this rest happens for you, soak it in. During this period, your baby will begin moving down into your pelvis without your even having to push, until an intense pressure produces an urge to bear down. This is called "laboring down" and is advantageous for both you and your baby, as it allows you both to recoup your energy. Laboring down also helps promote a vaginal delivery and can reduce perineal tearing.

When you do begin pushing, remember, descent is gradual: As your baby's head moves down with each push and contraction, it also slides back up during the rest periods. Interestingly, the force of your contractions will shift to the top of your uterus, as this incredible muscle helps inch your baby down and out. This stage can fly by in a few minutes or test your endurance over many hours.

Pushing and delivery is characterized by:

- Contractions lasting approximately sixty to ninety seconds

- Contractions that are approximately three to five minutes apart

- Dilation of 10 centimeters

- Complete effacement

Spontaneous or Directed?

Once your baby's head has descended to a low enough point, it will put pressure on a set of nerves called the Ferguson Plexus. This interaction triggers the Ferguson reflex, which is what causes the body to bear down and push with each contraction. In most cases, spontaneous pushing—that is, pushing only when you feel the urge—is effective, healthy, and satisfying for the mother. Yet in some cases, such as with the use of an epidural, your instinct to push becomes inhibited. In that case, those supporting you can direct you when and how to breathe, when and for how long to push, and when and for how long to relax.

So, What's Happening in Labor?

It's still unclear to scientists and doctors what gets labor started, but what is clear is that when it does, oxytocin is the primary hormone responsible for stimulating contractions. Influenced by the descent of your baby into your pelvis and the pressure its weight creates on your cervix, oxytocin is released on a positive feedback loop until your baby is in your arms.

Here's a quick guide on how your body and your baby keep things moving in labor:

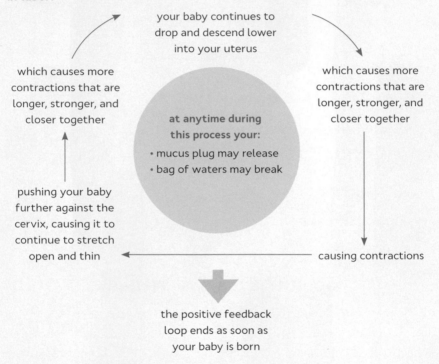

your baby continues to drop and descend lower into your uterus

which causes more contractions that are longer, stronger, and closer together

which causes more contractions that are longer, stronger, and closer together

at anytime during this process your:
• mucus plug may release
• bag of waters may break

pushing your baby further against the cervix, causing it to continue to stretch open and thin

causing contractions

the positive feedback loop ends as soon as your baby is born

Oxytocin flows best in labor if you . . .

- Feel safe, supported, and comfortable

- Use massage and movement and stay upright, allowing gravity to help you

- Use aromatherapy

- Remove distractions, such as unwelcome people or noise

- Turn down the lights

Contractions feel: As strong as they've ever felt, or stronger, but it feels really good to push as you're contracting.

Common feelings and sensations: Rectal pressure (you feel you need to have a bowel movement, but nothing comes out when you attempt to go); a burst of renewed energy; tingling or burning sensation at the vagina as your baby crowns.

Comfort measures: Relax your thighs and focus on bearing down through your hips, vagina, perineum, and butt. Seriously: Imagine that you're trying to gently force a flow of urine or a bowel movement—those are the muscles you're looking to engage as you bear down. Relax and rebuild between contractions; rest, and don't push if so instructed by your care provider (all pauses will help you regain strength for the next round and protect your perineum from tearing). Once your baby is crowning (head emerging from your vagina), ask to touch the top of his head or see a mirror—this motivation might just be the best antidote to pain and fatigue you've had yet. To minimize tearing, you should be encouraged to push gently, and your provider should provide counterpressure on your perineum, apply mineral oil around your baby's head, and help stretch your perineum and facilitate a more gentle delivery.

A note for your partner: If the mother asks for directed pushing, you may be called upon to count, coach, and encourage her in the moment. She may become animated while pushing or she may not, so it's best to stay in the moment, relax, and react to her cues. Try to be encouraging, stay positive, and reach deep into your motivational toolbox.

An Extra Push

If your baby needs a little help getting out, a vacuum extractor, forceps, or an episiotomy may be used to help assist.

Vacuum

A vacuum extractor is designed to support your pushes by keeping your baby from slipping back in between pushes. A cup lined with soft foam is placed against the crown of your baby's head. Pressure is generated by your care provider, using a handheld pump or by a nurse pumping from an external source. Traction is applied only during contractions, and you will be encouraged to continue bearing down as much as possible. It's usually abandoned if the suction cup slips off more than three times or if the procedure lasts more than twenty minutes. There are some risks to your baby with this procedure, such as bruising, scalp lacerations, and bleeding in the brain, all of which are rare.

Forceps

Forceps look like curved salad tongs. Each side of the forceps must be slipped separately into your birth canal around your baby's head. Forceps can help pull your baby out; they are also used to rotate the head to a better position for delivery. A numbing injection is applied if you're delivering without an epidural. Use of forceps presents an increased risk of perineal tearing.

Episiotomy

An episiotomy is a cut made in the back of the vagina to enlarge the opening for delivery. Episiotomies are not standard procedure, and if you'd prefer to avoid one, it's important to state this clearly; your wishes should be respected unless there is a medically urgent need to hurry the birth. An episiotomy offers no advantages over the spontaneous tissue tears that may occur during birth. The chance of tearing can be reduced with guided delivery, by your care provider applying supportive pressure to the perineum while your baby is crowning. In addition, warm compresses and mineral oil are also effective to guide your baby's delivery and to help minimize tearing. This is something to discuss with your care provider— ask how she handles care of the perineum.

Placental (Third Stage)

At this point, your baby will be in your arms after much hard work. The placenta is typically delivered within ten to thirty minutes after your baby arrives. You'll hardly notice this happening, as your placenta detaches naturally from the wall of your uterus. The delivery of the placenta is managed by your care provider, who may massage your uterus and gently tug your baby's umbilical cord to help the process along.

Common feelings and sensations: Severe shaking and shivering after your placenta is delivered is a common symptom and not a cause for concern.

Comfort measures: Take deep breaths and snuggle with your baby, especially when your uterus is being massaged. If your birth is unmedicated, this can feel pretty painful; it could be on par with a contraction in early labor.

To Eat or Not to Eat— A Common Placenta Question

Consuming the placenta or placenta encapsulation (having it dried and put into capsules) has become a popular choice for new mothers. There is little scientific research to support the largely positive anecdotal benefits; however, many women report they think it helped them tremendously postpartum.

Potential benefits are:

- Increase in oxytocin to help you bond with your baby and help your uterus shrink back down to your prepregnancy state.

- Decrease in postpartum mood disorders.

- Increased iron levels in the blood.

- Increase in milk production.

>>>

If you do decide to consume the placenta in a smoothie or in capsules, make sure to discuss it in advance with your care provider. She might have a referral for a local placenta encapsulator, or if you're working with a doula, she might offer that service. If you're birthing in a hospital, your doctor will need to sign a release to allow you take the placenta home. Also, make sure to bring a cooler box with you to transport it.

INTERVENTIONS

I don't think I've met a mother yet who didn't want an uncomplicated birth, where labor begins and progresses of its own accord. It certainly sounds great! Of course, that's what your body wants as well, and it's what's best. However, bodies are not cookie-cutter, nor are births. Your birth may have to be managed by the use of interventions, which can be offered to help start your labor, keep it on track, or ensure the safety of you and your baby. Let's explore some of the most common interventions that may come into play.

Inductions

Induction of labor means that your doctor or midwife causes your labor to start instead of waiting for it to begin on its own (see Hospital Induction Methods, page 225). Unless there is a distinct medical reason to rush the birth, waiting for labor to start on its own is the best choice for both you and your baby. In the U.S., the elective induction rate is on the rise, which means that inductions are increasingly being used in situations in which it is medically unnecessary. Remember, most first-time mothers deliver a few days to sometimes even a week after their due date, so it's not unreasonable to ask your care provider for more time and to work together on a plan to make that happen, whether it means more prenatal appointments or monitoring of your baby to make sure that all is well. Let's first review out-of-hospital methods that can help get labor started, followed by hospital methods, reasons why an induction might be medically right for you, and questions to ask if you think it's not.

Out-of-Hospital Induction Methods

Acupuncture and Acupressure

Acupuncture is the traditional Chinese medicinal practice of inserting thin needles into points along your body's meridian system (or life-energy paths), which are believed to influence specific organs or body parts. Acupressure, introduced earlier, is a lesser-known technique that takes advantage of the same points, applying physical pressure instead of inserting needles. Certain points can be stimulated to help encourage labor. For more tips on how to prepare your body for labor, see the guide on page 428.

Chiropractic

Some chiropractors use a labor induction technique at forty weeks combining chiropractic adjustments that stimulate the parasympathetic nervous system, activation of acupuncture points that ripen the cervix, and manual therapy to relax the ligaments around the uterus and pelvis.

Sex

Semen contains prostaglandins, which can help the cervix soften. Plus, orgasms release oxytocin, which can help promote contractions. Don't be surprised if your care provider tells you to go home and get busy.

Clary Sage Oil

While clary sage should be avoided during pregnancy, once you're at full term, it can be a gentle induction method. A few drops in a diffuser or about ten drops in a warm bath can help promote contractions.

Hospital Induction Methods

Induction of labor performed in the hospital is very common in U.S. obstetric practice when labor does not begin on its own, or your OB/GYN determines that it's safe for you and your baby if you deliver before your due date. About 40 percent of births are induced by either medication (e.g., Pitocin) or mechanical augmentation (e.g., rupturing the amniotic sac).

That said, inductions are not always the ideal option, particularly in the hospital. It's important to know exactly why an induction is being offered to you, as having an induction is associated with further interventions and even a higher chance of having a cesarean birth. These are the medical reasons an induction might be offered to you:

- Your amniotic sac has broken, but contractions have not begun after six to eight hours.

- Your pregnancy is "post dates" (forty-two weeks or beyond).

- Your amniotic fluid is low; this is assessed via ultrasound.

- You have a health problem, such as high blood pressure, pre-eclampsia (characterized by both high blood pressure and protein in the urine), or gestational diabetes, that can be treated only once your baby is born.

- You have chorioamnionitis, a bacterial infection of the two (amnion and chorion) amniotic sac membranes.

- Your baby has a problem that can best be treated after birth.

- Your baby has some problem that needs specialists present for the birth.

If these reasons are not given as the basis for your induction, ask these questions:

- Is there a clear medical reason for an induction?

- What are the risks of induction for my baby and me?

- What are the benefits for my baby and me?

- What method of induction would be recommended?

- What would happen if we decided not to induce labor? What protocol would I need to follow to have more time?

The induction options available to you will be determined by your provider based on the week of pregnancy you're in and how ready or "ripe" your cervix is. Your doctor or midwife will determine your Bishop score—a numerical score based on cervical dilation and effacement, and your baby's pelvic station. What follows are a few of the most common induction methods used by doctors and midwives.

Prostaglandin Medicines

Prostaglandins are hormones that help the cervix efface—thin and soften and get ready for labor. Synthetic prostaglandins (e.g. misoprostol) are placed behind the cervix during a vaginal exam by your doctor or midwife to soften the cervix to prepare it for dilation. Unlike previous vaginal exams, this one won't take place in your provider's office. Synthetic prostaglandins must be administered in the hospital where you will remain until your baby is delivered. The two main prostaglandin medications used in the U.S. are Cytotec (a pill) and Cervidil (a wafer-like insert). Cytotec's dosage can be increased every four hours, whereas Cervidil is given once every twelve hours, making it a better choice for some. Sometimes the medicine is put in place the night before the induction is to begin so that the mother can sleep while her cervix is getting ready. However, sleep might be challenging, as this procedure can be painful and result in moderate to strong cramping as the medication starts to work.

Stripping of the Membranes

During a vaginal exam, your doctor or midwife provider inserts a finger between the amniotic sac (amniotic membranes) and the cervix to loosen the membranes from the lower part of the uterus. This short procedure can be painful and cause intense cramping. This loosening irritates the uterus and helps your body release prostaglandins, which will promote contractions and help start your labor.

Artificial Rupture of Membranes (AROM)

Your doctor or midwife makes a small hole in your amniotic sac (amniotic membranes) during a vaginal exam. This is done using a special instrument called an amniohook. There is usually little discomfort with this procedure, but the contractions that follow will be much more intense. This procedure can be performed at a birth center or in your home if you're working with a midwife; if working with an OB/GYN in the hospital, you'll remain in the hospital until you deliver.

Foley Bulb

Your care provider inserts a Foley catheter (a slender rubber tube with an inflatable balloon at the end) through the vagina into the cervix and then inflates it with about 12 tablespoons [180 ml] of sterile saline. Your cervix must first already be dilated by at least 1 centimeter. The inflated balloon applies pressure to the cervix, which helps it open and dilate. When the cervix opens to 4 centimeters, the catheter will slide out on its own, and labor may start without any medicine. This procedure can be done at home with a midwife or at the hospital with an OB/GYN and can cause intense cramping and lead to strong contractions.

Pitocin

Oxytocin is a natural hormone in a woman's body that helps start labor, and Pitocin is a synthetic version used to emulate the hormone's natural effect. This drug is given through an IV by your doctor if your cervix has already softened and thinned considerably. Pitocin is typically started on a low dosage and slowly increased until the uterus begins to contract on its own. You may be able to request that you stop receiving Pitocin if your uterus is able to contract on its own. Contractions caused by Pitocin can go one of two ways: strong very quickly or a slower progression. Using options from the Comfort Menu (page 241), whether unmedicated or medicated, might be helpful. Because Pitocin can be a strong drug, its effects on you and your baby must be watched very carefully. If you are induced with Pitocin, you and the baby will be electronically monitored for all of your labor, and your movement may be limited. IV fluids will keep you hydrated and maintain blood pressure. You also will have a restricted diet of clear liquids in case you need further interventions that require an empty stomach, like a cesarean. Other risks include hyperstimulation of the uterus (meaning more than five contractions in ten minutes or individual contractions lasting more than ninety seconds), fetal distress in labor, and emergency cesarean. Nevertheless, when used prudently, Pitocin can be very useful, helping get your labor started or helping move it along if it's slowed down, and resulting in a successful vaginal delivery, if your cervix is ripe and ready to be induced.

When Pitocin might be offered to you:

- Approaching forty-two weeks of pregnancy, your cervix is soft and slightly dilated, but you haven't had any contractions.

- Your amniotic sac has ruptured, but after six to eight hours you have yet to have a contraction.

- An epidural has resulted in a slowdown of the labor process.

- Keep in mind that most medical inductions are a long game; think twelve to twenty-four hours of being at the hospital before your labor actually begins. If you are having an induction, consider working with a doula and having a game plan for finding comfort and balancing your rest and activity throughout the process.

CESAREAN BIRTH

As I've mentioned, and I strongly believe, all birth is natural, and a cesarean birth is no exception. That said, it does carry more risks for you and your baby than vaginal birth does, and increased discomfort during recovery. I've supported many clients over the years who have consciously selected this option or have had to choose it for medical reasons. Whether or not this is your chosen birth experience, there is a strong chance you might have one. As of 2013, the cesarean rate in the U.S. is 32.7 percent. So take some time to explore and understand this option, no matter what your birth preference may be. In the following section, you'll find information about why c-sections are performed, how they happen, and ways you can work with the experience to still have the positive, empowering birth story you envisioned for yourself.

Why Cesareans Happen

While there are many reasons a cesarean becomes medically necessary, from fetal distress to a breech position, there are also some nonmedical and non-emergency reasons you could encounter that might be more to the benefit of your doctor's schedule than to best serve you or your baby. Be sure to get a full understanding of the reasoning behind your cesarean from your doctor. By this point in the book, I hope you feel empowered to ask questions—and to decline an intervention (or at least seek a second opinion) if something feels off to you when a care provider recommends a cesarean.

Here are some typical reasons for a cesarean delivery:

- Failure to progress

- Breech position

- Fetal distress

- Hypertension

- Active herpes outbreak

- Placenta previa (placenta covers cervical opening)

- Prolapsed umbilical cord

- Cephalopelvic disproportion (baby's head too large for the pelvic opening)

- Emergency during labor

If a cesarean is suggested, consider asking:

- Is there a medical reason for a caesarean?

- What are the risks for my baby and me?

- What are the benefits for my baby and me?

What Happens During a Cesarean Birth

A cesarean section, or c-section, is a means of delivery whereby an obstetrician makes an incision into the mother's abdomen and uterus to surgically remove the baby. Typically, the mother is awake for the surgery and her partner is present for it. Traditionally, the cesarean incision was made vertically, from the navel to the pubic bone; however, the incision is now primarily done horizontally, below the belly and above the pubic bone. This incision reduces the risk of scar tissue rupture in the case of another pregnancy.

To prep for surgery, your pubic hair will be shaved (only near the incision site, not between your legs) and a catheter inserted into your bladder to keep it empty. Your abdomen will be washed in antiseptic solution and surrounded with sterile drapes. If you wish not to see the operation, a screen can be placed between you and your belly. Let your doctor know ahead of time if you would like for them to describe what they're doing or not. Doctors are generally aware of and used to both of these requests.

You'll be given an epidural, either spinal or general anesthetic (the latter is currently rare in c-sections). Once you are numb, incisions are made into your abdomen and your uterus. Your doctor will break your bag of waters, if it has not already ruptured; if you are conscious, you will hear a whoosh as the amniotic fluid is vacuumed away. Then the doctor will use their hands to push on your abdomen to ease your baby through the surgical opening. You will feel lots of pressure but no pain, and at this stage, you may be able to watch the birth happening, if you wish. (If you have a horizontal incision, you will not see anything too gruesome anatomy-wise.) Finally, your baby will emerge. The doctor will clear the baby's lungs and, once he's breathing, hand him to you or your partner. This entire process takes only ten to fifteen minutes.

Once your baby is born, you will be given an injection of Pitocin to help stop the placenta from shredding. Your doctor will surgically remove your placenta. Then it will be extracted through the incision. The doctor will stitch up the uterus and then your abdominal wall.

How to Make a C-Section Your Own

Family-centered or gentle c-sections, where there is less emphasis on traditional surgical rituals and an increased focus on facilitating the early interaction between you and your baby, are slowly becoming the standard of care. A family-centered cesarean celebrates the birth event and encourages early mother and baby bonding. What follows are some ways you can ensure a supportive cesarean experience.

Prior to Surgery

- If you cannot be conscious, ask that your partner hold the baby skin to skin immediately after birth, barring any medical complications with baby.

- Request that your anesthesiologist use nondrowsy medications, so that you can be as present as possible.

- So as not to interfere with breastfeeding, request that the blood pressure cuff be placed on your nondominant arm and the EKG placed on your back.

- If you'd like to have music playing, create a playlist for the operating room.

During Surgery

- Have a doula or another support person in the room with you.

- Ask if a clear drape can be used during surgery, allowing you to see when your baby is born.

- Have your gown lowered and your baby placed on your chest for skin-to-skin contact while you're being sutured.

After Delivery

- Ask to have your voice (or your partner's) be the first your baby hears after delivery.

- Breastfeed immediately, while in the operating room.

- Request a clamp delay until the umbilical cord stops pulsing. Sometimes this might not be possible, as your doctor may need to prioritize completing your surgery.

- Ask that you and your baby remain together in the recovery room to facilitate bonding.

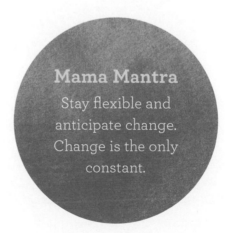

Mama Mantra
Stay flexible and anticipate change. Change is the only constant.

CHAPTER TEN

Finding Comfort During Labor and Building Your Birthing Preferences

Now that you know a little—OK, a lot—about labor and delivery, you likely have quite a few questions, maybe even worries, about pain management. You're in luck: I have more than a few great answers. In fact, this chapter really represents the nuts and bolts of my practice, or any doula's practice. Unlike a midwife or doctor, for the doula knowledge of birth and its inner workings comes second. For us, and for me, it's all about providing moment-to-moment support for the mother.

What follows is a culmination of my personal knowledge of what can truly help and uplift during labor. You'll learn some of the techniques I've found most effective: how to find your rhythm, make adjustments to find comfort, and follow through to an empowering delivery.

FINDING COMFORT DURING LABOR

Labor doesn't have the best reputation. In fact, you may have even stifled a little laugh when you read this section heading. The idea of being comfortable during or between contractions may seem idealistic or simply not a reality. Yes, it's true, labor pains are so-called for a reason. And yet, working alongside their bodies, I've seen my share of laboring mothers find relief; partners grow closer through these techniques; and mothers find strength testing the limits of their tolerance. You can do it, too.

Exploring Pain

First, let's think through pain and your relationship to it. Equal parts mental and physical, pain is interesting. Have you experienced significant physical pain? If so, what can you remember about it? What feelings are evoked when you think about it? Try to put yourself back in the moment of pain: What did you do or think about to find comfort?

Here's the thing with labor: The pain is different from and unlike any pain you've felt before. In the past, when you've experienced pain, it's been a response to random, uncomfortable stimuli, and maybe it's stuck around for weeks or months, like back pain or a sprained ankle. In labor, the pain you experience is finite (when your uterus is not contracting, you're not in pain), and it's bringing you closer to meeting your baby. It's purposeful pain, which might make how you navigate it different or give you more tolerance than you might usually have for pain and discomfort.

So what makes labor painful, anyway?

- The stretching of the cervix as it dilates, and the pressure of your baby on your cervix

- The stretching of your pelvic floor and vaginal tissues during the birth

- Buildup of lactic acid from the intermittent oxygen shortage to your uterine muscles when they contract (again, the pain disappears when the contraction stops)

The following lists can help you clarify your relationship to pain. Take each to heart and reflect: How do I best cope with pain? What can I do to prepare—both mentally and in my environment—to best move through pain? At the end of the exercise, review your lists, and share them with your partner and care provider so they'll have a good idea of how to move through your pain along with you.

Pain: A Deeper Dive

I'd like to encourage you to consider reframing how you explore the physical pain associated with labor versus pain in everyday life. They are innately different and this difference might help you with pain management during labor.

Physical Pain in Labor Is or Can Feel	Physical Pain in Everyday Life Is or Can Feel
expected—you have a due date, although the exact date is unknown, and you know that within a certain timeline, you will be experiencing some kind of pain due to labor	**unexpected**—you don't wake up expecting to be in pain, pain usually catches you by surprise, unless you suffer from chronic long-term pain due to illness or injury
purposeful—there is logic that supports it, this pain is bringing your baby into the world, and this is a reward that can make it easier to accept	**purposeless or inconvenient**—it can be hard to find the logic behind pain you are experiencing because there is no trade-off or reward to make it easier to accept
intermittent or noncontinuous—contractions come and go, allowing you to rest and have a break in between, when you're not contracting you should feel no pain	**continuous**—there might be no break from the pain, you could feel it all day and all night for days, weeks, or months as a result of an illness or injury
finite—it will come to an end when your baby is born	**like the end point is unclear**—you might not know when the pain will subside or end

What's My Comfort Level? A Checklist

(Check all that apply.)

When stressed or scared, I might . . .

○ Feel tension in these parts of my body:

_____

_____

○ Get a headache

○ Struggle to form sentences

○ Clench my jaw

○ Clench my fists

○ Cry

○ Fidget

○ Feel nauseous

○ Feel itchy

○ Feel my heart racing

○ Battle to breathe

○ Sweat

○ Bite my nails

○ Hear ringing in my ears

○ Other

_____

_____

_____

_____

I can stay calm if I . . .

○ Keep moving

○ Take a nap

○ Talk about what's going on

○ Change the environment

○ Be alone

○ Be with people

○ Express myself

○ Be touched or massaged

○ Meditate

○ Breathe deeply

○ Make a loud or silly noise

○ Listen to music

○ Have someone distract me

○ Analyze my thoughts

○ Work things out on my own

○ Seek advice

○ Eat a good meal

○ Take a bath

○ Other

_____

THE COMFORT MENU: VISUALIZATION

Visualization can help a great deal during labor, reducing stress, anxiety, and tension; decreasing pain; lowering blood pressure; and improving oxygenation throughout your body and your baby's body. Over the years, I've learned that visualization exercises should be simple; if they are not, they need to be guided. Listening to an audio track of guided visualization can help shift your mental state and mood. Apps such as Calm and Headspace provide a number of excellent options. Both guided and self-directed visualizations can help you rewire negative thought patterns. For example, if you find yourself thinking about how much the contractions hurt and questioning how you're going to get through it, visualizations can move you from focusing on "When's the next contraction?" or "Is everything OK with my baby?" into positive affirmations: You can do this, you are capable, and you and your baby are safe. Visualizations can help you collect your thoughts if your labor is tough or moving in a challenging direction, too.

Visualizations can also help you reap the benefits of your body's inherent pharmacy: It will release endorphins in response to pain. When your body comes under stress or experiences pain, neurochemicals called endorphins are produced in the brain's hypothalamus and pituitary glands. Endorphins, which are structurally similar to the drug morphine, are considered natural painkillers because they activate opioid receptors in the brain that help minimize discomfort. They can also help bring about feelings of euphoria and general well-being.

During visualization, breathe deeply. Your focused breathing will allow the mind to go offline, allowing your body's physiology to move into cruise control, letting you reap the benefits of the endorphin release. When you're tense and bracing and thinking about the last contraction and what's to come, your body stays stuck in fight-or-flight mode, blocking its ability to abundantly create or release endorphins.

I suggest using visualization as a reset between contractions. During contractions, use breath work and movement to ground and expand with the contraction. As soon as your contraction subsides, move into a visualization.

The key with visualizations is to practice, practice, practice. Try to begin your practice at the start of your third trimester. Aim to practice your visualization at least two to three times per week.

Self-Directed Visualization

Resourcing

This visualization is to help promote self-love, relaxation, and peace. You'll visualize four pleasurable and happy scenes from your past, followed by imagining four present positive happenings in your body. This visualization combines visual, auditory, and kinesthetic (touch) imagery. It's simple and effective.

The Steps

Take three deep breaths into your belly and let your body begin to relax.

Close your eyes, take another deep breath, and allow the relaxation to deepen.

Touch your thumb to your index finger, think of the easy feeling you have right before you fall asleep, let your body be loose.

Touch your thumb to your middle finger, think of the best hug or loving touch you've ever received, feel the touch through your body.

Touch your thumb to your ring finger, think of the sweetest compliment you've ever received, hear it right now, listen, and accept the compliment.

Touch your thumb to your pinkie finger, visit the most beautiful place you've every been, your spot. Notice the temperature there, the warmth or coolness, the quality of the light, the smells. Stay there for a while and take a nice deep breath.

BEGIN AGAIN

Touch your thumb to your index finger, allow your pelvic floor to relax, breathe down through your belly.

Touch your thumb to your middle finger, imagine your cervix opening and making space for your baby to descend into your pelvis.

Touch your thumb to your ring finger, imagine a warm pink light connecting your heart to your baby's heart. Take a breath to nourish yourself with that love; feel it pulsating.

Touch your thumb to your pinkie finger, think about holding your baby in your arms, stay with this feeling for a while, and breathe into your belly.

REPEAT

Visualizing your body opening and relaxing can empower you and make you feel like an active participant in your labor even as you relax. Remember, labor isn't just happening to you—you're helping it along, and you and your baby are working together toward a common goal.

The Safe Spot

This visualization is all about about creating a blissful place where you take your mind for a restorative break. Imagine an outdoor place where you can feel calm, peaceful, and safe. It may be a place you've been to before, somewhere you've dreamt about going to, or maybe a place you've glimpsed in a picture.

The Steps

Take three deep breaths, then tighten every muscle in your body. Hold for one breath, exhale, and relax your whole body. Take a deep breath and release it.

Begin to focus on what you can see in your safe spot. Notice colors, shapes, movement, light, and texture. Notice the sounds and the smells.

Now focus on any skin sensations: the ground beneath you, the temperature, any movement of air, anything else you can touch or that is touching you. Linger here a while, enjoying the calm and serenity that your safe spot brings. You can leave whenever you want to, just by opening your eyes and being aware of your surroundings.

While in your safe spot place, you might choose to give it a name—one word or a phrase that you can use to bring back that image anytime you need to.

THE COMFORT MENU: UNMEDICATED AND MEDICATED OPTIONS

What follows are the most common medicated comfort measures and interventions, as well as ample unmedicated ways to find respite as well. Review them well before labor and keep this with you—or with whomever will be there to support you—for reference. Find what works for you, in the moment. You may find a certain position does the trick every time or that you need to vary your methods hour by hour. Whatever the case may be, there are plenty of options available for you, mama.

It's Said and Done

Consult this handy acronym, **AFTER**, to figure out what you want to do about medicating.

- **Availability:** What does your birth environment provide?

- **Feeling:** How do you want to feel during labor?

- **Tolerance:** How do you handle and feel about pain?

- **Effectiveness:** How much pain relief do the available methods provide?

- **Risks:** What are the risks?

Medicated Comfort Measures

Your decision whether to medicate during birth can feel polarizing, but don't forget: It's your birth. Your body will progress as it needs to, and your mind will follow along, as well. React, adjust, and find comfort in the way that best suits you and only you. Remember, there's a difference between purposeful pain and unnecessary suffering, and it's important that you create pockets of ease in your birth experience so you're able to enjoy it. If you have a low pain threshold or any past trauma connected to pain, an epidural when you are ready might help you do just that. Know your limit, and know when to ask for help. Remember, soon you'll have to care for your newborn baby—do what you need to do for yourself today in order to be up to the task for her tomorrow.

Epidurals

Generally speaking, an epidural is any anesthetic injected into the epidural space (more on this shortly) that produces a loss of sensation from the waist down. They are the most popular form of pain relief during labor for a couple of reasons. Epidurals are local anesthesia, rather than a narcotic painkiller administered through an IV, and are therefore less likely to cross the placental barrier and affect your baby. The laboring mother stays alert and "herself" while using this drug, and yet can get enough pain relief to even get some sleep before delivery. There are several different types of epidurals available for laboring mothers, each with its own distinct features and benefits.

Walking Epidural

A lower dose than the traditional epidural, a walking epidural allows a mother more control and connectivity to her contractions. You will still feel your contractions, but not to the degree that you would without an epidural. Additionally, you will likely still be able to use your legs; depending on the liability parameters of the hospital, you may be able and permitted to move freely during labor.

Standard Epidural

A concentrated dose of anesthesia is administered by way of an epidural catheter, a flexible tube that an anesthesiologist inserts into the fluid in the epidural space, which is within the spinal canal but outside the spinal fluid. Once it's securely in place, you will be given a constant flow of the medication for the duration of your labor; you will likely have the ability to increase your dosage in the event of any "breakthrough" pain. This enables you to manage your pain with a relatively low amount of the drug, which should lessen side effects. Additionally, using less of the drug will give you a better chance to slightly feel your contractions, which should allow you to push more effectively.

Spinal Block

Also called a "saddle block," the spinal block is mainly used in assisted delivery, such as a c-section. A large amount of anesthesia is administered to the spine in a single dose, resulting in a complete loss of both feeling and muscular control below the waist. For this reason, this is not used in situations where the mother would need to push for delivery.

Keep in Mind . . .

- An epidural birth is not a wireless birth; you'll be hooked up, constantly monitored, and you'll be confined to a hospital bed.

- In 2014, the American Society of Anesthesiologists analyzed data from more than eighty thousand women who received epidural or spinal anesthesia during childbirth and found that the overall rate of complications was just under 3 percent. Complications include: nerve damage, permanent immobility (very rare), low blood pressure, loss of bladder control, itchy skin, headaches.

- A fever or low blood pressure can occur, becoming more likely the longer the epidural is in place, which can affect your baby's heart rate and oxygen level. It's generally not recommended to use an epidural before the cervix is 5 centimeters dilated.

- An epidural can prolong your labor by forty to ninety minutes, due to a decrease in your ability or urge to push.

Helpful Tips

- Ask for your epidural not once you've hit the wall, pain-wise, but when you feel you can handle only another ten contractions (or about ten to twenty minutes). It can take a while to gather the necessary practitioners, and the drug can take twenty to thirty minutes to become fully effective. A predetermined "safe word" can be helpful to alert your partner or doula that you are truly ready! The point is to avoid accidentally requesting an epidural in the throes of particularly challenging contractions when you may not have really wanted it.

- Try to relax. If you are tense or fearful, it can make getting the epidural more challenging. Having your partner or doula support you during the procedure can help keep you calm. Sometimes hospital policy limits the number of people in the room when an epidural is administered; ask your care provider what's possible beforehand.

- Epidurals work by gravity; if you begin to experience break-through pain on the uppermost side of your body, ask to be rotated onto that side; this will allow the medication to balance out, relieving the pain.

- You can ask for a lower amount of the epidural in the second stage of labor, which can help increase your sensation and the effectiveness of your pushing.

- Waiting to push until your baby's head is lower is called "laboring down" and can increase the feeling or effectiveness of pushing when you do begin. (It also helps prevent you from getting tired out.)

- You'll be on a limited diet with an epidural, but popsicles, broth, and ice chips should be allowed and can help keep you going.

You May Feel . . .

- Itchiness

- Breakthrough pain (areas on the leg or abdomen that are not fully numb)

- More numbness on one side than the other

- A headache

- Nausea

Back It Up

Here is how an epidural procedure goes:

- While seated, you'll be asked to arch your back like a cat while the anesthesiologist locates the correct place. The area will be washed and a numbing agent will be administered.

- The anesthesiologist will insert the epidural needle, then the flexible catheter tubing that will remain in your spine to continually administer the drug.

- The tubing will be taped down to prevent its being bumped or moved, and the drug will begin to flow.

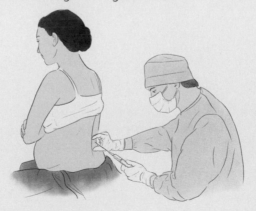

Epidural procedure

Know Your Lingo: Epidural Edition

Epidural catheter: An epidural catheter is secured in the epidural space in the spine so that the anesthetic can be continually administered. This allows for a smaller dose of the medication to be used, as opposed to a general anesthesia in the bloodstream.

Bladder catheter: Because a standard (nonwalking) epidural means no muscular control from the waist down, a bladder catheter is necessary to keep your bladder emptied.

IV drip: This is a flexible catheter attached to a hollow needle placed in your vein (usually in your hand or lower arm) to drip in fluids and medication. The needle is removed once the catheter is placed. This is typically a precaution to help prevent dehydration, but during an epidural, an IV is used to prevent a drop in blood pressure. Your hospital will insert an IV drip before placing the epidural (if they haven't required the IV upon your admission to Labor and Delivery, which is the policy at some hospitals). Hospitals can also require an IV drip during an epidural, because with the loss of sensation, the labor process typically requires some extra help with the drug Pitocin, which is administered intravenously. If you are not already planning on an epidural, a good compromise to strike with providers in the hospital is a saline lock—an intravenous (IV) catheter that is threaded into a vein via a needle, flushed with saline, and then capped off for later use. This way you are not hooked up to an IV pole, but the nurses have easy access in case you need medication later. Many hospitals require a saline lock for safety reasons.

Oximeter: Placed on your left index finger, the oximeter measures your pulse. This device is not necessarily in place for the entirety of your labor.

Blood pressure cuff: With an epidural, you will be constantly hooked up to blood pressure monitoring to ensure your pressure doesn't drop, a known risk.

External monitoring: Electronic fetal monitors are attached to two elastic belts that you'll wear on your belly during labor. One monitors the baby's heartbeat; the other monitors the frequency of your contractions. With an epidural, you'll wear the belts for the duration of your labor; however, you should check to see if your hospital offers remote (wireless) telemetry monitors, which are portable and will enable you to keep moving (if you opt for a walking epidural, for instance). If you're not using an epidural, your care practitioner will still need to monitor you, but it can be done intermittently instead of continually. Alternatively, your OB or midwife might use a fetal Doppler—a handheld ultrasound machine that uses sound waves to pick up and monitor your baby's heart rate and your belly while you're having a contraction to determine the strength of your contractions. This approach can feel less invasive and is standard practice at a birth center or home birth, but you can request it in the hospital as well. Try not to focus intently on the monitor data itself; that information is for your care providers to assess. Tune in to your body and baby and how you're coping; that will help you stay centered.

Internal monitoring: If there is a reason to suspect fetal distress, or your doctor would like to be able to more accurately monitor your baby's state, internal monitoring may be suggested or required. This is a small electrode inserted through the vagina that measures the baby's heartbeat. Contractions are monitored internally with an intrauterine pressure catheter, inserted through the vagina into the amniotic space. Though internal monitoring gives a slightly more accurate record of these data points than an external monitor, it's used only when absolutely necessary because it comes with a higher risk of infection.

Other Common Medicated Comfort Measures

In terms of medicated comfort, epidurals are the preferred intervention. There are, however, many different pain relief medications available, one of which may turn out to be a good option for you. The following table presents some of the most common meds available.

What It Is	What It Does	Possible Side Effects
Nitrous oxide	Commonly known as laughing gas, nitrous doesn't interfere with labor and isn't a pain-killer. You'll still feel your labor and contractions, but you'll feel indifferent to the pain. Used very widely in Europe and a growing number of hospitals and birth centers in the United States.	Side effects are very minimal. You breathe the gas in through a mask and have control of dosing. It's very difficult to become over-sedated; however, if this happens, nausea can occur.
Tranquilizer	Curbs anxiety and nervousness, especially if those feelings are interfering with the progression of labor (as a result of the production of the stress hormone cortisol).	Depending on dosage, it could make you feel sleepy or even fall completely asleep.
Demerol, (or other intravenous narcotics)	A painkiller, Demerol will curb the pain felt from delivery. It can also be used to regulate the rhythm of contractions.	Sleepiness, nausea, and vomiting are common. As with tranquilizers, the risk of side effects is transferred to your baby as well.
General anesthesia	Renders the patient unconscious for the entirety of the birth. Extremely rare for birth these days; used only in cases of extreme emergency.	Considered fairly safe, although you and your baby would feel groggy afterward. You will also not be present (alert, awake) for the birth.

Unmedicated Comfort Measures

Whether or not you're planning to incorporate some type of medicated support into your labor and birth, I urge you to internalize the following sections detailing unmedicated comfort measures. These techniques are useful and important for any birth, whether it's an epidural birth in a hospital, a nitrous birth in a birthing center, or an unmedicated birth at home. Giving birth is a profoundly significant episode in the life of any woman; it's a time when we reach for support from loved ones, reach emotional limits in all directions, and find previously unknown inner strength. What follows are some truly effective methods to help you out.

Here's What to Do

Simply put, this is how you labor:

Keep it loose. Follow your body's cues and go with the flow.

Use gravity. Try to stay upright, using a yoga ball, birth bar (a bed attachment that helps facilitate squatting and other positions), or partner for support.

Move. It might seem like a tall order, but getting up and moving helps mitigate pain.

Speak up. Always express yourself if something isn't working or doesn't feel right.

Rest. Between contractions and whenever you can.

Hydrate. Support your effort by taking in fluids.

THE COMFORT MENU: NOURISHMENT

You may have heard that eating and drinking during labor isn't possible or will be restricted, but actually you should be encouraged to nourish yourself during labor, especially an unmedicated one. Eating will help you feel normal and healthy and assist you in meeting the rigorous demands of labor. In fact, being undernourished may be associated with longer and more uncomfortable labor.

Typically, birth centers will allow you to eat and drink freely while you labor there. Hospitals are more variable. Some may not allow you to eat, due to their internal policies; others may allow it. There was more concern in the 1940s, when women were typically placed under general anesthesia to give birth, and eating introduced the risk of vomit being aspirated into the mother's lungs. With a spinal block or epidural, this really shouldn't be a concern—aspirating food or drink while under anesthesia is statistically less likely than being struck by lightning. Have a frank discussion with your care provider if you feel you're clashing with your hospital's policies.

Early Labor

Graze and fill up on food that will fuel you for several hours. You will more than likely still be at home and can take advantage of your own kitchen. Aim for light, well-balanced snacks or a meal that includes complex carbohydrates, with some protein and healthy fat to stabilize blood sugar and energy. I love these options:

- Avocado toast

- Hard-boiled egg

- Oatmeal with honey and butter

- Yogurt or some hard cheese

- Banana or apple with nut butter

- A protein smoothie

- Dates

Active Labor

Many women naturally self-regulate their food intake during labor, eating and drinking less as their labor picks up and intensifies. Don't be surprised if you find you are not that hungry later in your labor. If you are hungry, try these options:

- Honey, especially convenient honey sticks

- Applesauce

- Rice cakes

- Bone broth

- An electrolyte drink (make your own by combining 4 cups [960 ml] coconut water, ¼ teaspoon sea salt, 1 teaspoon calcium magnesium powder, and 1 tablespoon honey)

- Frozen ice cubes of Nettle Raspberry Infusion (recipe on page 98)

THE COMFORT MENU: BREATH

I like to think of the breath as your conveyor belt during labor: It keeps things running, and if it gets stuck, chances are you won't be running well either. Unless we're being consciously asked to pay attention to our breath, as in a yoga class or during meditation, we tend to take it for granted. During labor, it's essential to stay mindful of your breath and to take care to breathe with intention.

There are many different theories of labor breathing, but there is no definitive one. Whatever is comfortable and effective for you is the best breathing technique for your labor. If all else fails, do what keeps your face loose and your jaw relaxed (more on why that's important shortly). What follows is a basic rundown of different breathing techniques for labor. Try them and see which ones help you ride through each contraction more easily.

The Sigh

When a contraction begins, take a deep sigh. Drop your shoulders and release any tension as you exhale. Take your next breath in through your nose and exhale with another big sigh. This is great way to begin a contraction because it will help focus your energy to begin breathing, focusing, and relaxing. It will also signal to your partner and other birth support that you have started a contraction so they can offer their support as well.

Early Breath

During early labor, when contractions are less severe but beginning to build, you'll still be able to talk through your contractions. Since the pain isn't quite as intense, this is a great time to start practicing and committing to memory the techniques that might be a little tough to remember once the pain increases. Try this:

- Start with the Sigh.

- Relax your jaw as you breathe by whispering "la la la" to yourself.

- Slowly breathe in through your mouth to a count of four, then out through your mouth for another four.

- Exhale like you're blowing on a feather: light and easy.

Active Breath

During the active phase of labor, contractions are strong and at times can feel overpowering. You will not be able to talk through them, but you will be able to breathe through them very effectively. Try this:

- Start with the Sigh.

- Breathe in slowly through your nose to a count of two and out through your nose for a count of two, breathing from your belly, not your chest.

- When exhaling through your nose, blow out slow and strong.

- Keep your jaw relaxed by slightly separating your lips.

- If you have trouble breathing through your nose, feel free to breathe through your mouth.

Pushing Breath

For the main event, you're going to pivot your breathing technique away from relaxation and internal motivation, and start focusing your breath on uplifting your energy and getting that baby out! Pushing is a high-energy period of labor, and your breath can help motivate you through it. I like to think of this breath as one that "turbocharges" each contraction. Try this:

- Start with the Sigh.

- Inhale deeply and hold that breath in the back of your throat (not your cheeks) as you bear down and push for five to ten seconds. Relax your jaw and the muscles in your face; you want that fiery breathing energy extending to your belly and bottom, not tensing up your facial muscles.

- Continuing to bear down, exhale, then take a quick, deep inhalation and repeat. Continue in this pattern for as long as the contraction lasts.

- If your baby is crowning or you have the urge to push, but you're being told to slow down, try to pant, pant, blow. As you blow, remember the feather image again and imagine blowing it far away.

How Your Jaw Affects Your Labor

Have you ever felt hip pain from an injury in your hamstrings? Or noticed that your neck began to hurt from low-back strain? Muscles relate to and affect each other throughout your body, and the muscles associated with birth are no different. When you have a contraction, the abdominals pull up on the pelvic floor and pull down on the chest, which pulls on the neck, which pulls on the jaw. With every contraction, remember that the tension from a contraction isn't just in your belly; paying some attention to releasing your jaw muscles can significantly help alleviate the tension of contractions, which in part can help your cervix relax and open. Try the following exercises during and in between contractions and notice how they can affect tension.

- Mouth the letters A, E, I, O, U as wide as you can, using the full range of motion in your jaw.

- Relaxing your lips, blow air through them, making a sound like a motorboat. This is a great de-stressor during strong contractions.

- Slightly parting your lips, whisper the word "la" over and over; notice how your jaw relaxes.

- Sounding, or vocal toning, is a practice used by singers to warm up the singing apparatus: diaphragm, vocal cords, throat, and facial muscles. When used in childbirth, it helps relax the abdomen and the perineum as well. Think low, vibratory sounds, like "mmmmmm" or "ohhhhhhhh" (both of which are impossible to make with a tight jaw!).

THE COMFORT MENU: MOVEMENT

Moving during labor is important. In fact, unless you've chosen to get a nonwalking epidural or have received specific instructions from your care providers, there is no reason to labor in bed the entire time. That said, you'll find that many of the exercises here translate well to the bed. Movement helps reduce pain, encourages your baby to rotate, and engages gravity to draw your baby down and keep your baby pressed against your cervix, which creates the necessary pressure to help it thin and open. The strongest and most effective contractions happen when your baby's head is well engaged with your cervix.

The movements in this section are meant to be used in a dynamic circuit, much like circuit training in the gym. I chose the word "circuit" intentionally because unmedicated labor is a workout—maybe the ultimate workout. The largest and strongest muscle in your body, your uterus is working hard to release your baby into the world. As your labor intensifies, you might need help to keep moving; this is where your partner or doula can be of great help. Begin practicing the circuit at least six weeks before your due date so you and your partner and/or doula become comfortable with each move. Think of it as training; once a week is ideal. This will also help relieve any aches and pains you might be experiencing toward the end of your pregnancy.

Get a Move On

Consider the following gear for your labor circuit.

Birth Ball

The birth ball (as we'll now call it) is a traditional exercise ball used in physiotherapy and fitness environments. It's more comfortable than a chair and allows for mobility; you can sit, lean, or kneel over the ball during labor. The upward curve of the ball provides support and takes the strain off the lower back and sacrum. Swaying forward and back during contractions can be a big pain buster.

Select a birth ball based on your height:

- 55 cm: under 5'4" [1.63 m]

- 65 cm: 5'4" to 5'10" [1.63 to 1.79 m]

- 75 cm: over 5'10" [1.79 m]

When sitting on the correct size ball, your knees should be level with your bottom or form a 90-degree angle. If your bottom is higher than your knees, the ball is too big or it's overinflated. If your bottom is lower than your knees, it's either too small or underinflated, which narrows the pelvic opening, creating less space for your baby to make her way through the birth canal.

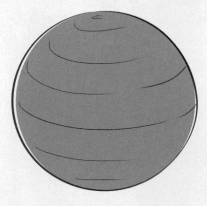

Birth ball

Peanut Ball

The peanut ball is a modified exercise ball. Less well known than the birth ball, it's gaining popularity because it can be used if you're confined to bed, making it helpful if you have an epidural or complications, or are just plain exhausted. When placed between your legs, the peanut ball opens the pelvis and the pelvic outlet, helping your baby rotate and descend more easily.

Select a peanut ball based on your height:

- 40 cm: under 5'4" [1.63 m]

- 50 cm: 5'4" to 5'10" [1.63 to 1.79 m]

- 60 cm: over 5'10" [1.79 m]

Inflate your ball until it feels firm, and make sure that it can rest comfortably between your legs.

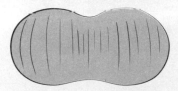

Peanut ball

The Movement Circuit

The goal with the movement circuit is to move into a different position every thirty to forty-five minutes or every five to ten contractions. This constant change will help you manage the pain with each contraction, help your baby rotate, and employ gravity. The trick with movement is to start it as soon as you feel a contraction start to build and continue to move until the contraction is over. If you try to begin moving at the peak of your contraction, it will be difficult and you won't realize the full relief potential.

Balance out your activity with rest. When you're not having a contraction, stand still, walk slowly, sit, or lie down. Energy conservation is key during labor. I've seen many labors move from unmedicated to medicated not because the pain is overwhelming, but because the mother was simply too tired. Food and hydration are critical as well, so graze as you go.

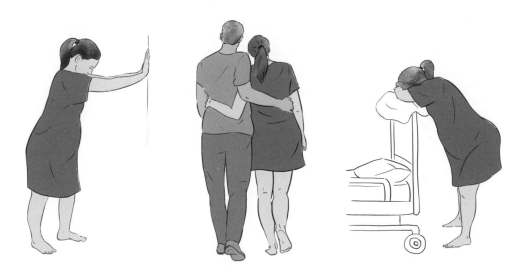

Demonstration of Walk, Stop, and Sway

Walk, Stop, and Sway

Some women like the sense of control they get from standing and walking during active labor. During contractions, you can stop to lean against the wall or on your partner. When you do stop, spread your legs hip-distance apart, to make space for your baby to descend, and sway gently from side to side. You can also lean over a table and sway.

Squat and Sway

Squatting benefits both you and your baby. It relieves back pain and can help speed the progress of labor by relaxing the pelvic and perineal muscles and engaging gravity. Squatting gives your baby a straighter route through a wider passage, creating the easiest path for moving through your pelvis. You can squat against the side of your bed or, with the support of your birth ball, against a wall, or you can just lean your back against a wall.

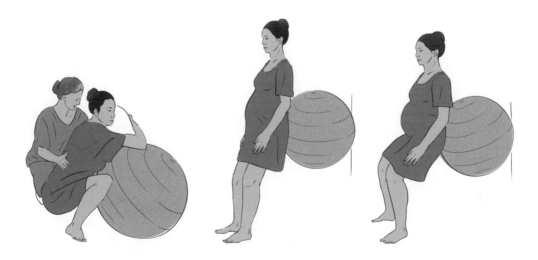

Demonstration of Squat and Sway

Ball Circles

Sitting upright on a birth ball, open your legs hip-distance apart so that you can sit comfortably without feeling wobbly. Sway your hips from side to side, then round and round. You can also have your partner or doula sit in front of you in another chair; you can lean into them while you circle round and round, providing more comfort.

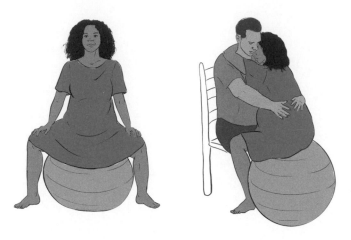

Demonstration of Ball Circles

Rock It Out

Rest your upper body and head on the ball. You should be able to lay your left or right ear down comfortably. Make sure your knees are open hip-distance apart. Roll forward on the ball, then backward, bringing your bottom all the way to the ground in between your knees. For a variation, extend one leg out into a bent position to the side of the ball and rock in and out, opening up your pelvis. This can feel tight and uncomfortable, and one side might be more open than the other; use your breath to move through it. The more you do it, the easier it will get.

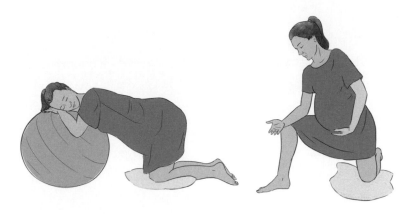

Demonstration of Rock It Out

The Tilt

Get down on your hands and knees, arms shoulder-width apart and knees hip-width apart, keeping your arms straight but not locking your elbows. Relax your back into a straight neutral position as you gently look upward, relaxing your neck. Then as you breathe in, tuck your buttocks under and round your back, trying to keep your belly loose. Relax your back into a straight neutral position as you breathe out. Repeat at your own pace, following the rhythm of your breath.

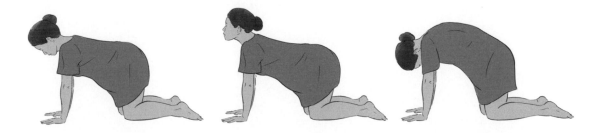

Demonstration of the Tilt

Open Knee Chest

Move from the Tilt position into Open Knee Chest by leaning forward and folding your arms together, then resting your head down in between your arms, making sure your chest is on the ground. You can sway your behind as you rest and turn your head side to side for comfort. This position helps reduce early labor back pain; if your baby is posterior (facing toward your pubic bone rather than your sacrum), this can move him into a better position.

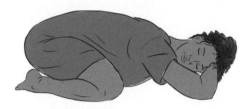

Demonstration of Open Knee Chest

Active Rest

Lie on your right side, right hip and lower leg straight, and left hip and knee bent. Place a pillow in between your knees. Although you're lying down and rebooting, the Active Rest position helps your baby rotate and keeps your pelvic outlet propped open, making space for the baby to descend, and increases blood flow to the uterus. This effective position can feel uncomfortable, especially during a contraction, as your baby descends. For relief, pair it with the Press and Tilt massage (page 271): have your partner place a hand on your sacrum and, as you tilt your hips out, press the whole weight of the hand against your sacrum, creating resistance. Rest here for a few contractions and switch to your right side.

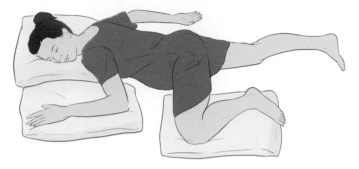

Demonstration of Active Rest

Sitting on the Toilet

This position is in the movement circuit for two reasons. For one, it's a reminder to go to the bathroom. Having an empty bladder and bowels makes more space in the abdominal cavity, allowing more space for the uterus to contract effectively. Sitting on the toilet can also help automatically relax your pelvic floor muscles and perineum. Why? Because you're used to doing that when you sit on the toilet, in order to release waste—there's already a built-in association. This position also opens your legs and creates and uses pelvic pressure, helping you dilate and open. Plus, when you have a contraction in this position, rocking your hips forward and back is very effective in helping decrease your discomfort.

Hydrotherapy

Hydrotherapy relaxes the muscles, provides comfort, and reduces the production of stress-related hormones. By reducing anxiety, it also can increase the release of oxytocin and endorphins, helping you dilate and contract. If you're birthing at home or a birthing center, you can incorporate hydrotherapy by getting in a bath or birthing tub (with water no warmer than your own body temperature) while you labor and deliver. In the hospital you can sit on your birth ball or stool in the shower and let the water stream over your back. The best time to use hydrotherapy is during active labor, when the contractions are most intense.

Epidural Circuit

This circuit was developed to accommodate the limited range of motion that comes with an epidural. The focus here is to incorporate some movement, keep your pelvis open, and help your baby rotate and descend. These two positions have been shown to help promote vaginal delivery and reduce the need for further interventions beyond the epidural. Your nurse, partner, and/or doula will assist you in getting into these positions. Try to change position every two hours; that way you can get some rest in between.

Active Rest with Peanut Ball

Lie on your left side, left hip and lower leg straight, and right hip and knee bent. Then place your peanut ball between your knees. This pose can be started on either side. You should change sides every 1 to 2 hours to help your baby rotate and descend. Although you're lying down and rebooting, Active Rest helps your baby rotate and keeps your pelvic outlet propped open, making space for your baby to descend. You won't feel any discomfort, but if you still have some mobility you can do the Press and Tilt massage, tilting your hips in and out (just like the pelvic tilt) against the pressure being applied to your low back. This flexion and extension can help your baby descend. Have your partner be mindful of hand placement when doing this massage; be careful to avoid where the epidural has been placed.

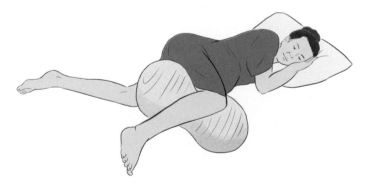

Demonstration of Active Rest with peanut ball

The Throne

Sitting semi-upright with one leg over the peanut ball and another leg open to the side can help keep your pelvis open, making room for your baby to rotate; this can help reduce the length of your labor. This position can allow you to feel more active in the birthing process when your mobility is limited. Switch legs every thirty minutes.

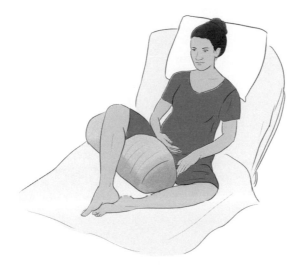

Demonstration of the Throne

THE COMFORT MENU: MASSAGE

Try weaving some massage throughout your labor, cycling among movement, rest, and massage as coping methods. Massage can be relaxing and calming, and can also provide much-needed counterpressure to general bodily discomfort and the pain of contractions. What's more, you simply can't massage yourself in the places where you really need it in labor, so these exercises can be a great source of connection for you and your partner. Your partner will likely feel proud and more fulfilled by being able to be an active support in your labor.

Many of the discomforts that these massage techniques address are not unique to labor—you may already be experiencing back and hip pain as early as six months in. Ask your partner to try these moves in the months leading up to delivery day, especially those last uncomfortable weeks as you wait for your baby.

Partner Massage Tips

Ask where she likes to be touched. It's important to know what areas might be off limits, and always ask for permission before you start any massage.

During contractions, no news is good news. Try not to ask how a massage stroke feels during a contraction; it's best not to distract her. No feedback usually means "all is well, continue with what you're doing." She'll let you know if it doesn't feel good or if she needs more or less pressure.

Stroke with intention, in the same direction. Long mid-pressure strokes, using the palms of your hands, work best.

Get warm. You can use hot compresses or packs to provide more relief; this works particularly well on the shoulders and sacrum. They should have them in your hospital or birth center, or you can make them by soaking a washcloth in hot water.

Avoid applying pressure to the bones and joints.

Source and Release

This practice is great for the end of your pregnancy, to help you become more receptive to receiving touch, and also to understand where and why you might be holding tension in certain areas during your labor. Ideally, with this exercise, you can train your mind and body over time to relax in the area being touched. Blend this practice with your desired breathwork.

Before birth, try this exercise:

Before your partner or doula touches an area of your body, mentally and physically create tension there. As they touch the spot, release into their touch and let the tension melt.

During birth, you can take this exercise one step further to release specific areas of tension in the moment. Here are some common examples of areas that hold tension during birth and some exercises to experiment with before the big day.

Belly: During your contractions your abdominal muscles tense up, making your breath more shallow and increasing your pain. Light pressure just above your pubic bone can help ease pain and tension.

Try before: Tense your belly, and as your partner touches your pubic area, relax that area.

Shoulders: You'll probably find during the first stage of labor that you tighten your shoulders during contractions. This can lead to tight, shallow breathing, which decreases the oxygen that your baby receives. Slow, firm pressure on your shoulders can help release this tension.

Try before: Tense your shoulders and have your partner rest both hands over your shoulders, pressing down slowly and firmly.

Head and face: During labor you'll tend to tighten your facial muscles, especially around your eyes, forehead, and jaw, especially if you're anxious or focusing hard. This tightening stiffens your jaw, which will make it more difficult for you to release your pelvic floor. If your jaw is tight, you're clenching throughout your body, holding on to tension.

>>>

Try before: Tense your face. Your partner can massage your temples and then your jaw just below your earlobes to encourage you to let that tension float out of your face.

Arms: During a contraction you will probably find that you clench your hands, creating tension throughout your arms.

Try before: Tense your arm. Your partner can gently touch your clenched fist, encouraging you to open it, and then move their hand up the inside of your arm to encourage relaxation throughout.

Legs: As your baby descends and presses down, there's a chance that you will tighten the muscles of your legs, particularly in your inner thighs, and maybe try to close your legs. It's important to keep your legs open and your inner thighs loose and relaxed to allow your baby to travel down easily.

Try before: Tense your legs. Your partner can help release this tension by placing one hand on the inside of your thigh and the other hand on the outer side of your thigh, and gently gliding and molding down your leg to your ankle.

Pelvic floor: Your pelvic floor will tighten as your baby's head moves into your vagina; learning to relax this area now can be helpful.

Try before: Try pulling your pelvic floor upward, tensing it like you're trying to holding in pee, to the count of three. Then, as your partner touches your inner thigh, release your pelvic floor downward to the count of three until you can feel your vagina begin to slightly bulge.

Buttocks: During labor, tightening your buttocks is a common response to the intensity of your contractions. However, when you tighten your buttocks you also tighten your pelvic floor, making it harder for your baby to descend. Your partner can help you keep your buttocks loose by firmly massaging them, as you would knead pizza dough.

Try before: Tighten your buttocks, then as your partner begins to massage them, release the tension.

The Massage Circuit

For Partners: Neck and Shoulders

Make a soft (loose) fist and, using the base of your hand, apply pressure on her left shoulder. Run your hand up the side of her neck until you get to the base of her skull, then go back down. Without breaking contact, repeat on the other side. Do this a couple of times, especially during a contraction, as this technique will encourage her to relax her jaw.

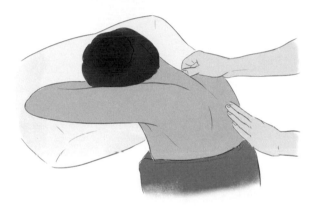

Demonstration of Neck and Shoulders

For Partners: K1

This acupressure point helps release the pain of contractions and pulls the energy in her body downward to calm stress. It's located at the center of the sole of the foot, two-thirds of the way up from the heel, just below the ball of the foot. Once you locate the point, press and hold it firmly. You can also press it on both feet at the same time.

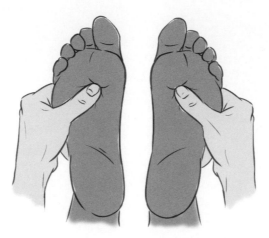

Demonstration of K1

For Partners: Hand Massage

To help soothe hands and arms, which can get tired from clenching, grasp her hands in your hands, placing your thumbs in her palms. Squeeze her hands, applying a good amount of pressure and increasing if she asks for it. Begin to move toward the fingers, squeezing with that same pressure as you go all the way down to her fingertips.

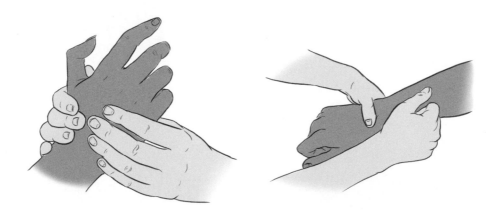

Demonstration of Hand Massage

Press and Tilt

Releasing pressure on the sacrum and thereby on the uterus can be extremely helpful in early labor or if contractions wake you up in the middle of the night. Lying on your left side, place a pillow or peanut ball in between your legs to help keep your pelvis open. Bend your knees, if that feels comfortable, or keep the leg beneath you straight and your top leg bent. Have your partner place their entire hand on your sacrum and, when a contraction begins, begin to tilt your pelvis backward and forward, like a cat stretching, picking up the pace if you need to. The faster you go, the more pain relief this massage will provide, so you can customize it. As you tilt back, your partner should push on your sacrum, creating resistance. This resistance helps release the low back and the ligaments around the uterus and the sacrum in order to create less pain during the contraction. Continue throughout the contraction.

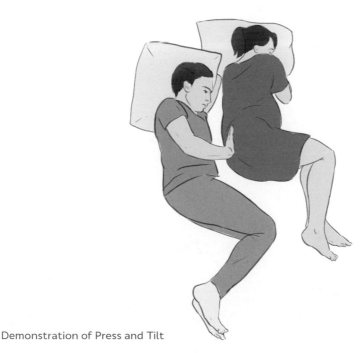

Demonstration of Press and Tilt

Hip Squeeze

The Hip Squeeze is a type of pressure massage that can relieve lower back pain in labor. It pushes the pelvis back into a more open position, relieving the pressure created by your baby moving through your pelvis.

Get on your hands and knees, leaning over your ball or a bed. Have your partner place their hands on your hip bones at the sides of your hips, then move down to the side of your buttocks. For proper placement their palms should be in the fleshy circle of the buttock muscle, not on any bone. They should then push into your buttocks toward the center of your body, squeezing your hips together. They can move around to find the exact right place to press—when they find it, it should not feel painful, but like a release. Have them steadily press it through each contraction with as much pressure as you need. Feel free to sway gently during the contraction as they squeeze. This technique can also be performed with a rebozo, a long piece of fabric that's been used in childbirth for centuries; it can help give your partner or doula a break but still give you the steady pressure you need. To do this, have your partner gather the rebozo under your belly and around the hips, and pull in opposite directions (pull one end of the fabric in left hand to the right side and vice versa). They can then add a knot in the fabric at your sacrum to keep it tight and then add more counterpressure on your back.

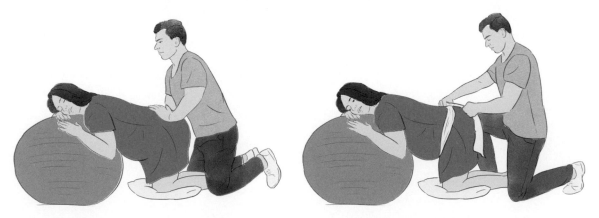

Demonstration of the Hip Squeeze

Abdominal Lift

Freestanding or against a wall, interlace your fingers and place them against your pubic bone underneath your belly, cradling your belly. During a contraction, gently lift your abdomen up and slightly in toward your spine about 1 to 2 inches [2.5 to 5 cm] while bending your knees. As you bend your knees, you can begin to sway from side to side. Before labor you can do this if you are feeling a lot of abdominal pressure, and as you become more comfortable you can do it freestanding without a wall.

During labor this should help take pressure off of your low back and make a contraction more bearable. If you have a nurse or midwife with you, it is a good idea to ask them to check your baby's heartbeat while doing the abdominal lift to make sure that no pressure is being placed on the umbilical cord.

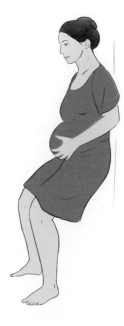

Demonstration of the Abdominal Lift

Ready, Set, Release

You can boost endorphins, promote relaxation, and foster more effective contractions by moving through these steps in between contractions.

- Release the upper body with a shoulder massage.

- Release facial tension by opening your mouth wide or with a jaw massage.

- Release the lower body by having your partner jiggle each leg.

- Release your bladder; urinating frequently gives the uterus space to contract more effectively.

PUSHING POSSIBILITIES

OK, this is a big moment! You've been laboring for who knows how long. Maybe you've labored down and now your doctor or midwife sees that your baby is ready to make his big appearance. How you get him out will have a lot to do with his position, so listen to your body and your care providers to decide which methods feel most effective. Try pushing in several different positions. It may take some experimenting to find your bearings and get your rhythm, but once you do, pushing will start to feel liberating and bring you closer to officially meeting your baby.

Your baby follows a curved path when exiting your vagina, so when you bear down, you'll want to imagine you're pushing down and then slightly forward in the shape of a J (rather than straight down). Prior to labor you can practice the sensation of pushing. While urinating, gently try to push the flow of urine down and forward. When you're having a bowel movement, try to create gentle and precise pressure down and curved toward your back. Building this association will aid you when you're pushing in real time; even if you have an epidural, this early association will help you conjure up the acuity of those muscles from memory.

Oh, and about pooping in labor: Look, it might happen. You're using all the right muscles. In fact, most women do poop during labor. Don't stress about it—it's nothing your birth team hasn't seen before, and they'll clean you up with warm water and gauze or a clean towel. If you're nervous about your partner getting a full view of that action, ask them to stay up north, looking into your eyes and helping to motivate your pushes.

Pushing Pointers

Curl around your baby, like a ball. This flexion will help your baby descend.

Tuck your chin. Right into your chest as you curl forward.

Use gravity. Try and stay in upright positions as much as possible.

Bear down quietly. Vocalizing during early and active labor can help move things along, but when you push you need all of your energy, and vocalizing during a push can reduce the energy you're putting into bearing down.

Think toilet. Yep, I said it: When bearing down, imagine that you're using the muscles that allow you to urinate and have a bowel movement. This awareness can help whether you're medicated or unmedicated.

Ask for direction. If you're struggling to feel exactly where you need to push, you can ask your care provider to insert their fingers into your vaginal opening and apply some gentle pressure to help you discern where to send your energy when you push. This can be helpful if you have an epidural.

Keep your legs open. As your baby descends and starts to crown, you might find yourself wanting to close your legs and resist her coming through, especially if you are unmedicated, as the feeling can be intense and you may instinctively back away from it, rather than pushing into or through it. However, closing your legs narrows your baby's passage and only makes it harder for her to make her way out. Your partner or doula can assist you in remembering to keep your legs open.

All Fours and Kneeling

Although pushing or giving birth in a kneeling position may be used by any woman, it may be especially effective if you have had back pain during labor, as it helps encourage movement of the baby. During the contraction, you tilt or curl your hips under and lower your buttocks slightly as you push. Between contractions, you can drape yourself over the head of the bed to rest and relax, or over your birth ball if your wrists become tired. Ask your partner or care provider to place a pillow or rolled-up hand towel under your feet and another behind your bent knees when using this position. The towels help your feet and legs relax and be more comfy if you're in this position for a long time.

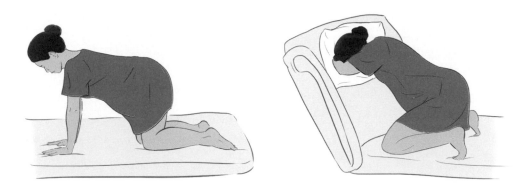

Demonstration of All Fours and Kneeling

Sitting Upright and Squatting

This upright sitting position is a variation on the use of a birthing stool. Notice how the mother is curled forward around her baby, with her elbows out as she pushes. The head of the bed is raised high, and the foot of the bed is lowered, giving you a place to place your feet. Like the use of the stool, this position helps you use gravity effectively. Between contractions, you can lean backward, supported by the bed. If you like, your partner can also sit behind you in bed as you use this position.

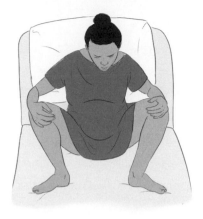

Demonstration of Sitting Upright and Squatting

Side-Lying

Side-lying is a preferred birth position for lying down, as it doesn't put pressure on your major arteries (and therefore doesn't inhibit blood flow to the baby), which can be the case with the lithotomy position (lying on the back with legs elevated, often in stirrups, as for a pelvic exam). Side-lying is also beneficial for instances when the birth is proceeding too quickly, or if you're laboring with an epidural or monitoring that prevents you from getting out of bed, or if you need a break and would like to lie down. It also leaves your back open for some labor massages from your partner or doula.

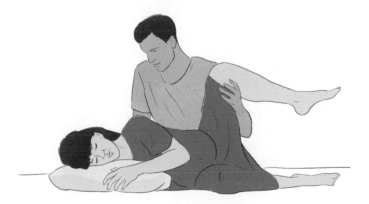

Demonstration of Side-Lying

Semi-Seated and Lithotomy

This position is not as effective in opening the pelvis as the upright positions illustrated earlier, but is probably the most common position used in a hospital for the actual delivery of a baby—not necessarily because it is the best position for birth but, as you can imagine, it is the most convenient position for your doctor or midwife. That said, I have seen many women enjoy and successfully push in this position, especially when it's one of many positions they choose to push in. In this position, the head of the bed is raised to at least 30 degrees or greater, and the mother can have a pillow placed under her right hip, helping her turn slightly to the left. These adjustments help keep the weight of her uterus and baby from interfering with blood flow. She can also curl forward around her baby, holding on behind her knees, and her support people can merely support her legs and her upper back, without pushing on them.

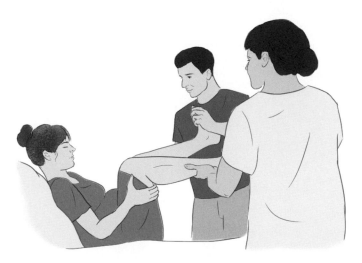

Demonstration of Semi-Seated and Lithotomy

On the Sunny Side

Generally speaking, back labor is any labor in which the laboring mother feels significant (read: extreme) pain in the lower back during and between contractions. When back labor is not present, you should get a break in between contractions and feel no pain at all. This is what makes back labor especially challenging: It doesn't provide a break. When doctors or midwives refer to back labor, however, they are almost always referring to a labor in which the baby is positioned "sunny side up," or in posterior position—that is, with her face pointed toward your belly rather than your rear. In birth, your baby makes a complicated series of twists through your pelvis before crowning, and with a posterior baby, extra pressure and force is put on your pelvic bones and sacrum as she attempts to fit through, well, facing the wrong way. A posterior position is more likely to happen in an induced birth or with an artificial rupture of the amniotic sac. Head back to Month Eight to read about what you can do during your pregnancy to help encourage your baby into the best possible position for birth and potentially avoid back labor altogether.

If you're experiencing back labor, try this:

Get into Active Rest position (pages 262–263) and change from side to side every hour or less. This can help shift your baby into a new position and take pressure off of your vena cava (a major interior vein responsible for returning deoxygenated blood to your heart).

Move around. Change positions every few contractions to encourage a last-minute flip from your baby and to keep pressure from settling on one particular spot. Open Knee Chest and the Tilt are especially effective.

Warm or cold. Alternate between warm and cold therapy. Ask your partner or labor support to apply heat packs, hot washcloths, or cold packs to your low back to relieve discomfort; this works well in between contractions.

Massage. The Press and Tilt and the Hip Squeeze can be great pain relievers for back labor; have your partner or labor support move into those as soon as a contraction begins, holding until it ends.

THE COMFORT MENU: AROMATHERAPY

If you're one of the many pregnant women whose sense of smell is heightened at this time, you know the power of scent. A certain odor can produce a visceral reaction, from calming, serenity, and well-being to revulsion, upheaval, and unrest. In this section, we'll talk about some of the best scents for fostering those good feelings.

While candles (at home), sprays, and other premixed scents are easy and certainly helpful, I love essential oils best. You can mix several to create a soothing custom blend, or use individually, for a potent energy boost. Here are my favorites:

- Clary sage: A uterine stimulant that promotes smooth contractions and provides pain relief. (Should not be used during pregnancy, only once you're in labor.)

- Lavender: Helps reduce anxiety and anger and manage stress.

- Frankincense: Helps ease anxiety, is grounding, and soothes restlessness.

- Geranium: Helps balance moods related to hormones.

- Peppermint: Energizing and awakening, great as a pick-me-up when you start to push.

The Essential Labor Blend

Makes 2 ounces

2-ounce [60-ml] glass bottle with
   pump top
1/3 cup [80 ml] almond oil
8 drops clary sage

5 drops lavender
5 drops frankincense
5 drops geranium

Add the oils to the bottle and swirl to combine. Massage the mixture into the skin as needed.

How to Use Essential Oils

Massage. You or your partner can use blended essential oils, like the Essential Labor Blend, for massages during labor. The heat created by the hands helps the oils penetrate through the skin and work to relax you.

Diffuse. Use one or two oils when diffusing. Clary sage and lavender work well together and are palatable to most noses, which is important, because everyone around you will be inhaling it too. An electric ceramic diffuser is the way to go; add three drops of each. This is a wonderful way to set the mood in your labor space.

Inhale. Put a few drops of each oil on a tissue paper, place it on your chest, and inhale deeply. You can also place the tissue paper underneath your pillowcase. This can be great in between contractions or if you have an epidural and are looking to soothe your stress and boost your energy. Another way to inhale the oils is in the shower or bath; place a few drops on the shower floor or in your bath, where the warm water will disperse the scent.

Mist. Making a hydrosol spray can be a great refresher, especially if you can't use a diffuser or need a break from massage. Get another 2-ounce [60-ml] spray bottle, add all of the Essential Labor Blend ingredients except the almond oil, and spray away. This can be great in between contractions.

The Postpartum Shift and Early Motherhood

Congratulations: You did it! You are officially a mother. Here's the thing: No matter how your birth went—dreamlike, easy, and fast or challenging, traumatic, and stressful—you are now on the other side. Here, there's so much room for growth. In Part Four, we'll look at what I call "the postpartum shift"—the first four weeks after having your baby. This period is one of transition, healing, and bonding.

Over the centuries and across cultures, the postpartum period tends to be a time when a mother's community surrounds her. She's taken care of; she's able to rest while someone looks after her baby. She does as little as possible while healing, typically within the first forty days. This is especially true in many Asian and South American traditions. In the United States, however, new mothers don't always get this level of support after birth. You might feel, as you're reading this, that you have to do so much of this on your own. I completely understand why that might feel overwhelming. It's not an easy job.

The most important thing about this period is to go slow, eat well, and rest often. You may experience the blissful surrealism that tends to characterize this moment, but it can also be a time of complex emotions and demands for rapid acclimation. Depending on who you are and how you've lived your life, you may be more equipped or less equipped to navigate it. These next few chapters will give you the information and skills you'll need—everything from baby care to relations with your partner—so that you can support yourself, heal quickly, and enjoy this time with your newly expanded family.

CHAPTER ELEVEN

The Recovery Path:

Helping Your Body Heal

————

So, yes, that really just happened: You carried a baby in your belly for nine months (give or take) and then gave birth! We have a lot to thank our bodies for; yours, for instance, just worked very, very hard and did something incredible. And today, it might not feel its best. In the first few weeks after birth, it can even feel that your body is no longer yours. It's different than it was before you became pregnant; you may be breastfeeding around the clock, feel like you have less control over certain bodily functions, and be just plain exhausted. And, what can feel the most disorienting, you may likely have some battle wounds: tears, blood, swelling, stitches.

Beyond your body, your mind may feel taxed and overwhelmed with new emotions as all those pregnancy hormones start to leave your system. Or you may be dealing with negotiating relationships with your family, friends, and even your partner. There's a lot to take in and sort through during these first few weeks of motherhood, and I'll help you do it. In this chapter, we're going to look at all these normal physiological events that might feel foreign and learn different transition smoothers to help make it easier for you to get back to being you.

YOUR BODY

On the day you give birth, you've spent the better part of a year slowly acclimating to your pregnant body. Little by little, your body grew, changed shape, and gained a new, previously unknown purpose and power. After delivery, with your baby now on the outside, your body might be somewhat unrecognizable—and it will be doing some things it's never done before, very suddenly and with little time for acclimation. Take this in and take it to heart: Your body is not broken. You might feel like you'll never be able to collect yourself and get back to normal. The opposite is true. Your body is on a very rapid healing trajectory, and you will be surprised how quickly some components bounce back; other areas might take a little bit longer. Here are all of the most common body changes you may (or may not!) have postpartum.

Exhaustion

You just completed the most intense physical event of your life, followed by a flood of the most powerful emotions you've ever felt. You're learning, in every moment, how to care for your new baby; compound this with a lack of consolidated sleep, and you're understandably exhausted. Here's some solace: This is all normal. As much as you can, try to embrace all of it. Try not to be hard on yourself or judgmental. Sometimes, accepting that you're supposed to be tired and that you will be tired can spare a new mother from feeling badly about it.

Here are a few transition smoothers for exhaustion:

Embrace the fatigue. It's OK to be tired. Don't expect yourself to be zipping around in the first couple of weeks. Acknowledging your limitations can bring some ease. Know this: The model of a super productive day for a new mom is feeding your baby, changing your baby, and sneaking in a nap.

Rest when your baby rests. Newborns sleep on average sixteen to eighteen hours per day, but not in long stretches. At the most, she'll sleep for a three- to four-hour stretch. For women who aren't used to taking naps, try what I call an "active chill time." Get horizontal, pop on a podcast or a guided meditation, or catch up on your favorite TV show, and allow your mind to wander and to be absorbed somewhere else.

Go to bed early. It's important to somewhat parent yourself at this time. Avoid the temptation to stay up to your previously normal hour—say, 11 o'clock. If you take an earlier bedtime, even 8:00 P.M., you won't feel as exhausted when you get up for a night feeding.

Lochia

The lochia is vaginal bleeding postpartum. It's how your body gets rid of the remainder of the uterine lining after birth. It will feel and look a lot like a period, although it has several different phases. For the first one to three days after delivery, the discharge will be a bright red color. Then it will turn a pinkish or brown color for the following week. From about ten to twelve days onward, you'll have more of a yellow or white vaginal discharge. The lochia can end at around two weeks or can last for up to six weeks. Clots will range from pea-size to grape-size. If you're frequently seeing clots larger than that, make sure to alert your care provider, as it may be a sign of a secondary hemorrhage. Don't be alarmed, though, if you see larger clots in the morning or when you get up after a nap—with gravity, the lochia may collect and coagulate.

Here are a few transition smoothers for lochia:

Depends—yes, the adult diapers—are great to have. I like them because you can just wear them. You don't have to worry about messing up your underwear; they're more streamlined (and generally less bulky) than high-absorbency maxi pads. They're also high-waisted, which helps to contain your postpartum belly a bit. Once the amount of bleeding begins to decrease, usually within a few days, you'll probably want to transition out of your original Depends. Go for their Silhouette range. I also love Thinx, a brand of underwear that actually absorbs period blood.

Eat iron-rich foods. Beets, bone broths, and grass-fed red meat are all helpful for recalibrating your system after birth and all the iron loss from the lochia. I really like Floradix, an excellent vegetable-based iron supplement that you can take on its own or add to a smoothie.

So-so sheets. Make your bed with a pair of sheets you're not super attached to. I have to say, Depends do a great job, but you may still experience some leakage due to the high volume of the lochia.

Swelling and Sweating

You've taken on a lot of extra fluid during your pregnancy to nourish your baby and his amniotic fluid. Additionally, after delivery, especially with a medicated or cesarean birth with extra IV fluids, many women are very swollen. What may start to happen immediately after your delivery is excessive, excessive sweating, called diaphoresis. This is how your body gets rid of the extra fluid that was built up over the course of your pregnancy. You'll experience what I call "your own private summer"—everyone else in a room is cold, and you're boiling hot and sweating. This can last for a full six weeks, so although it may be tempting to ignore it and just forge ahead, there's no need to be stoic; taking a few comfort measures can really help.

Here are a few transition smoothers for swelling and sweating:

Wear breathable (read: all natural) fabrics. You'll want your clothes to be loose and probably made of something in the cotton or linen family. Don't overlook your sheets: Switching those for lightweight linen can really help and allow you to sweat through.

Add a waterproof pad under your bedding to absorb extra sweat and protect your mattress.

Bodywork or a **massage** can work wonders for the circulation and also be a nice opportunity to sweat it out. No need to wait on this: Try to get a massage in the first week if possible.

Stay hydrated. You're losing so much water, it's important to make sure that you're replenishing the amount that your body needs to maintain. Keep water by your bedside.

Keep towels by your bedside. If you wake up sweaty, you can wipe off.

Urinary Issues

You may already have experienced some urinary issues before birth. Pregnancy hormones can trigger a reduction in muscle tone in the bladder and urethra. Add in an expanded belly bearing down on the whole system and an unfortunately familiar (and yes, very common) pattern might arise: laugh, then pee; sneeze, then pee; cough, then pee. It's called stress incontinence, and you can have it even if you have a cesarean birth. Postpartum that incontinence can continue and may be slightly more severe because of the pressure from delivery. Additionally, after delivery the sensation of needing to urinate can be reduced. You may have a full bladder, not realize it, then experience some incontinence. With this issue, be slow and forgiving with yourself—it can take a while to regain strength in the area. If by three months it hasn't resolved, look for a physical therapist specializing in women's health. They can provide toning exercises and internal massage to speed recovery.

Here are a few transition smoothers for urinary issues:

Go frequently. Simple enough, and yet, as noted, you may not have the necessary sensation. I even recommend setting an alarm on your phone. Make sure you're emptying your bladder at least every three hours to get back into the rhythm. Even if you don't feel like you have to, more than likely some urine will come out.

Depends, part two. Your Depends can help with more than just lochia. If you do happen to release some urine without knowing it, they'll clearly help.

Pelvic floor toning. If you are not already routinely doing your Kegels, exercises that tone your pelvic floor, it's time to start. Try an elevator-style movement with the same muscles you use to cut off the flow of urine, pulling in and up for the count of three, then releasing down for the count of three. Start as soon as it feels comfortable, which may take a bit of time, depending on your birth experience. When you are cleared for exercise, traditional Pilates can help, too.

Constipation

No matter what type of delivery you had, you will likely experience some constipation. In a vaginal birth, with all that strong pushing, the rectal and perineal area can feel very tender. If you've had a cesarean, your internal system will obviously take more of a hit from surgery; it can take up to seventy-two hours until you have your first bowel movement. The typical way we deal with constipation is to make sure that the stool is extremely soft and easy to pass. For this reason, a laxative is not preferred; a stool softener is. You will eventually have a bowel movement, so we want to make sure that it's as painless as possible when it does occur. Your care provider will offer you a stool softener, but if you aren't comfortable with that option, there are some gentler ways to approach it. That said, after a cesarean birth, the stool softener and dietary protocols set forth by your doctor are the best way to go.

Get on the Floor (Been So Long)

Pregnancy hormones softened and weakened your pelvic floor muscles, then birth stretched them as far as they could go. It's no wonder they'll need a little attention after birth (and once you're ready and comfortable). Here are two great ways to rehab the pelvic floor.

First, try bringing awareness and sensation back into the area. Lying on your back, pretend you're trying to prevent yourself from passing gas, contracting your anus. Relax, then pretend you're holding in urine, engaging your pelvic floor muscles. Relax, then try to contract the walls of your vagina. And relax. Try these as frequently as is comfortable. Don't worry about trying to hold these muscles for a long time or intensely; all you're doing at this point is locating and engaging. Even a second is helpful, and don't be worried if you can't do any of this at all. Keep trying. It will come with time.

Now let's make some space with your breath. Lying on your back, raise your arms over your head into a wide "V" shape. In this position, take a deep breath to open your ribs in the front and the back, and as you exhale, make a "Ssssss" sound. This helps open your rib cage and assists in deep breathing. Now let's go back in and get specific. Imagine your vagina partitioned into three sections: bottom, middle, and top. Staying with this deep breathing style, contract the bottom of your vagina for five seconds, then release it and relax. This should feel subtle. Then contract the middle of your vagina for five seconds, release, and relax; then contract the top, release, and relax. Try to practice these exercises once a day.

Here are a few transition smoothers for constipation:

- Psyllium husks mixed with water. Add ½ to 2 teaspoons psyllium seed to 1 cup [240 ml] warm water. Mix well and drink immediately before it becomes too thick to swallow comfortably. (Psyllium thickens rapidly when water is added to it.)

- Carrot juice.

- Prunes.

- Coconut oil, taken by mouth, 2 to 3 tablespoons.

- Digestive enzymes can also help ease digestion and promote more bowel movements; take them before a meal.

- Chelated magnesium (300 mg once a day).

The Pooch

Women are always surprised they still have a belly after delivery. Even if you worked out every day of your pregnancy, maintained muscle tone, and followed a perfectly healthy diet, you still just housed a baby for nine months. For at least the first month, there will be a significant pooch, but there are a couple of things you can do to help relieve the "loose" belly feeling you may be experiencing.

Here are a few transition smoothers for the Pooch:

Lie on your tummy. One of the best things you can do to help your belly go down is to rest on it. Literally—lying face down on your belly, resting your head on a pillow. This can provide a very gentle massage to your uterus, and encourage the organs and tissues that have shifted to move back into their natural place. A similar effect happens when you're lying on your back. Standing up, doing housework, being out, and doing too much too soon all subject the organs in your lower pelvis to a constant downward pull of gravity. When you lie down, the pelvic organs can settle and no longer press against the perineum, helping it heal more quickly. Try and give yourself at least a week before engaging in any major housework.

Belly binding is actually an ancient tradition that endures today. The modern form involves using an elastic fabric or corset-like top that you pull around your torso to help guide everything back into place. Belly binding isn't simply for vanity and a flat stomach, either; many women complain about feeling "uncollected," and belly binding helps offer great lower back support, which can make picking up and holding your baby and moving about feel easier. There are a number of different brands and options on the market. I like a neoprene waist trainer, typically used for exercising. It's made for comfort and movement, and the fabric is breathable and allows you to fasten the band quite snugly. See The Goods (page 422) for my specific recommendation. Aim to wear your chosen belly binder for a few hours a day, and always take it off to sleep.

Headaches

Headaches are very common after delivery, especially if you've had an epidural or spinal block. Even an unmedicated vaginal delivery can result in headaches simply from the next-level exertion that went into your labor. Add a lack of consolidated sleep and sweating that can easily lead to dehydration, and headaches are a near probability.

Here are a few transition smoothers for headaches:

Take medicine. Depending on the degree of your pain, something that may provide immediate relief is the fact that your baby is no longer inside of you, so now you can take any medication or herb recommended by your care provider that truly helps ease you. Ibuprofen is A-OK. (The amount that will get to your baby in breast milk is very, very small.)

Hydration is important due to the amount of sweating you'll be experiencing. Additionally, the production of breast milk requires lots of water (more on that in Chapter Twelve), so really make sure you're getting enough. Drink every time your baby drinks.

Inject caffeine. It's really OK to have a cup of coffee or tea to help dilate the blood vessels and relieve tension. Having a little bit of caffeine is not contraindicated with breastfeeding, and it can help ease your headache.

Hemorrhoids

Hemorrhoids are typically caused by a lack of motility in blood flow in the lower intestinal tract. For this reason, you may have already experienced hemorrhoids before giving birth, as progesterone slows the flow of blood throughout your intestinal tract. It's also common for women to experience them, either internally or externally, from pushing during birth as well. Hemorrhoids can be very uncomfortable and downright painful.

Here are a few transition smoothers for hemorrhoids:

Witch hazel pads offer topical support that can be helpful; this astringent helps draw the fluid back into the body. You can buy them already saturated. You can even leave one there directly on the hemorrhoids, with your Depends or underwear acting as a retainer.

A sitz bath is helpful if you're especially itchy and uncomfortable. It's essentially a small basin that fits in your toilet bowl, which you'll fill with warm water and a soothing herbal solution (usually some combination of lavender and calendula and plantain leaf; see page 296 for my blend).

A hemorrhoidal cream like Preparation H is also helpful after a sitz bath.

Try a medical procedure. If these methods aren't helpful, hemorrhoids can be lanced and removed. Don't hesitate to bring up any lasting or near-chronic pain or discomfort with your doctor.

Perineal Discomfort

Your perineum (the area of skin between your vagina and anus) bears a lot of the brunt from all your hard work pushing that baby out. Pressure from your baby's head, transferred down from the force of your contracting uterus, hits squarely in this region. Plus, it also stretches to accommodate your baby's head, which often leads to tearing. The overall sensation in this area after birth will be similar to rug burn. It will pass—remember, you're healing very quickly!—but until then, it can feel uncomfortable to do simple things like sit in a seat or on a toilet. Also, after a vaginal delivery you should avoid taking a full bath and submerging yourself in a tub until one week after birth (showers are OK) because your vagina is more vulnerable to infection. Opt for a sitz bath while you wait out this period (more on this follows).

Here are a few transition smoothers for perineal discomfort:

A peri bottle (perineal irrigation bottle) or bidet will help cool, soothe, and cleanse this area. This is especially important to do when you urinate in the early days post-pregnancy, as uric acid and sodium can sting when it touches open skin, and it can feel tender to wipe. Have your peri bottle in the bathroom, and as you pee, immediately spritz water from the bottle onto the tender area to help dilute the urine.

A sitz bath is useful for perineal discomfort as well, especially in the first twenty-four hours after delivery. Most have some sort of opening in the back to allow liquid to spill back into the toilet. If urinating is really stinging, try relieving yourself into the full sitz bath.

Take a warm bath. A few days after delivery, run yourself a warm bath with 1 to 2 cups [255 to 510 g] of Epsom salts stirred in.

Cold and warm therapy. In the first twenty-four hours, cold therapy from ice is fantastic for providing relief and reducing swelling. A latex glove filled with ice can be super convenient—and exactly the right size and shape. Take some from the hospital or birth center, or ask your midwife for a few to hold on to. After the first twenty-four hours, you'll want to move to warm therapy from a warm (not hot) compress to bring more blood to the tissue. You can do so in your sitz bath.

Try a donut cushion. These are wonderful for helping to take the pressure off of your perineum when you sit, as the weight of your body is evenly distributed around your buttocks. Take it with you from room to room. That said, if you're struggling to sit comfortably it's a sign that you should be lying down more—take that as a big hint.

Try a numbing spray such as benzocaine for severe pain. Use three to four times a day for the first week after delivery.

A Good Sitz

This sitz bath is easy to make and is a healing powerhouse to help repair and soothe the skin of your tender perineum. Plantain leaf has antimicrobial, anti-inflammatory properties. Calendula flower is also antimicrobial, helps reduce pain and inflammation, and is known for healing skin without leaving a scar.

....

Calendula and Plantain Sitz Bath

1 cup [300 g] sea salt

½ cup [170 g] dried calendula flowers

½ cup [170 g] dried plantain leaf

1 cotton muslin bag, 5 x 7 inches
   [12 x 17 cm]

4 cups [960 ml] boiling water

5 maxi pads (optional)

Combine the salt, calendula, and plantain in a medium bowl. Then scoop the mixture into the muslin bag and close. Place the bag in a large bowl and pour the boiling water over it. Allow to steep for 15 minutes. After steeping, take out the muslin bag and gently squeeze out the excess water. Pour the infused liquid into your sitz bath bowl. Sit in the mixture in your sitz bath bowl for at least 10 minutes and then air-dry your perineum.

Alternatives:

- Pour the liquid into your peri bottle and use it to rinse when you urinate in the first few days. It will keep for three days. After that, discard any unused liquid and make a fresh batch.

- Soak the maxi pads in the infusion and freeze them in a large zip-locked bag. Use them individually as needed in the first week to few weeks, if you need cold relief on your perineum. Place the pad inside your underwear for no more than 10 minutes.

....

Uterine Cramping

At delivery, your uterus was five times its normal size; after delivery it undergoes a process called involution to return to its former size. Almost immediately after you give birth, it will begin cramping and tightening (and expelling lochia in the process). The degree of pain or discomfort varies for different women. Some barely feel it or notice it, like a light pressure; others report it feeling like early labor cramps revisited. You'll notice it most when you're nursing, when the body releases oxytocin, which aids in both milk release and the contractions of involution.

Here are a few transition smoothers for uterine cramping:

Locate your uterus. First things first: Have your nurse or postpartum doula show you where your uterus is right after birth. That way, you can place a hand there and, right before you begin to breastfeed, gently massage the muscle so it won't be quite as tight if it starts to cramp up.

Warm compresses or an electric heating pad are also helpful—particularly when nursing.

Lying on your stomach will help the pooch and help cramping by applying pressure to the organs. For bonus relief, lie on your belly on a heating pad— but for no more than fifteen minutes.

Low Back Pain and Body Aches

You've just wrapped up the most intense physical event of your life; it makes sense that your entire body might be pretty sore, much like after a hard session at the gym. Low back ache is also common because your baby stretched your pelvic girdle, which puts extreme pressure on your sacrum and all the muscles in your low back. Add to this a lack of (or reassigned) core strength and the demands of lifting your baby, and you'll need some support.

Here are a few transition smoothers for low back pain and body aches:

Getting a massage the first week after delivery can help push out the lactic acid built up in your body from labor. Try to get an in-home massage if you can, so you don't have to leave the house. There are many on-demand massage apps now, so you can even squeeze one in during your baby's naps. Plus, if the massage is in your home, you can pause to tend to your baby if need be.

Try an infrared sauna session around week two or three for about fifteen to twenty minutes. Infrared saunas help your body sweat and relax, and can help relieve pain. They also help increase your circulation and purify your skin. Infrared saunas heat the surrounding air but to a lesser degree; their heaters emit a specific wavelength of infrared light. Your skin absorbs this wavelength, causing your body's temperature to rise. This creates the same effects as a traditional sauna with less overall heat needed, which is preferable and more comfortable for most. Make sure to drink a ton of water while you're there and after, especially if you're breastfeeding.

Cesarean Care

Even with a cesarean birth, you'll likely experience many of the symptoms just discussed. You'll also have several additional factors to deal with. If you've never had major surgery before, you may not know how to care for an incision or be familiar with the appropriate level of activity during recovery. Here are a few transition smoothers for after a cesarean birth:

- **Pain management:** You've just undergone major surgery, so you will be managing your pain with the use of prescription pain medication. After nine months of pregnancy with no medication, it can feel strange to start taking something right away, but in fact, the best thing is to take it as prescribed. The key is to take the medication before you feel discomfort or pain—typically every four hours, depending on the drug you're using.

- **Uterine cramping:** If you experience involution, the uterine cramping described earlier, try to relax all your muscles as much as possible. Resist the urge to tense up your muscles; lying limp and breathing in through your nose and out through your mouth while the cramping is taking hold can be helpful.

- **Mobility:** Within about four to six hours after your birth and every few hours after that, you're going to need to move around the hospital. In fact, the staff will encourage it. Movement helps with the healing process and circulation. You can also do exercises to promote circulation in bed. For example, with your legs outstretched, try pressing the back of each knee into the bed, one at a time. Make ankle circles; spell your baby's name with your toes.

- **Ask for help:** Your abdominal muscles need a big rest, so you may need support even for simple things like getting in and out of seats, picking up your baby, or opening a sliding door. Plan for someone to be there to assist you. Especially if you are on pain medication, you may feel upbeat, but it's important to be mindful and avoid lifting anything heavy.

>>>

- **Take it slow:** You won't be able to move very well or quickly after having a cesarean, so make sure to assess each physical situation you encounter, and be honest about what you can and can't do. If you have trouble getting into bed, getting on all fours can help. When standing up, it may help to keep your torso straight rather than leaning forward.

- **Gas:** Anesthesia slows bowel movements, so that function will be stalled for two to three days after delivery. This will likely create some gas. Drinking warm water with lemon can help, as well as the following movement (no pun intended): While lying in bed, stretch your leg outward with an exhale, then bend it with an inhale, resting your foot flat on the bed. Repeat slowly and gently on each side, four or five times.

- **The scar:** Your incision will take four to six weeks to fully heal, though it's not unusual to still feel pain at the incision site past that time. For the first couple of days after delivery you should not get the incision wet, so you won't be able to fully shower. A washcloth or sponge bath is a good option. Always make sure you wash your hands and dry them with a paper towel before you touch the bandage or that area. To aid healing, you can drink valerian root tea to help with swelling. Once you no longer need a bandage, vitamin E oil is great for hydrating the tissues and stimulating repair. Ask your doctor about scar-reducing creams or scar therapy.

YOUR MIND AND EMOTIONS

The hormonal surges and resulting emotional spirals you experienced during pregnancy are about to get a whole lot more complicated—and a lot more nuanced as well, as the cushy pregnancy hormones decrease (or rather, stop abruptly) and your own mental tendencies absorb and work through this momentous change.

Bonding

We've all heard these stories: "I fell in love immediately." "It was a strong feeling I had never had before." "As soon as my baby was in my arms, I truly knew what love was." Some women do, in fact, have these moments. Most think they should, though many don't—and that's very, very normal, although it's not as widely shared as the love stories. In my practice, I've heard many retellings of the first moments: It can also be bewildering, strange, alien, and even scary or intimidating to hold your baby for the first time. Further, we're not all built the same: For you, a true bond may come from caring for your baby over time or when he finally looks you in the eyes and smiles. No matter where you are in the spectrum, you can help deepen or move bonding forward with the help of a few of the following transition smoothers:

- After delivery, even if the connection doesn't feel immediate, looking into your baby's eyes, making eye contact, and simply gazing can help you take him in. Don't feel like you have to feel anything; just look at him and let your mind absorb him, signaling to your mind and body that this is real.

- Skin-to-skin contact has many health benefits, and it has emotional benefits as well—both for you and for your baby. Allowing your baby to rest on your bare chest can release a swell of oxytocin to facilitate the hormonal work of bonding.

- Lastly, bonding may just take time. Always be patient with yourself and your baby. It may just take a bit of time for you to acclimate and begin to feel the reality of your baby in order to bond. Give yourself time to warm up to her; it's absolutely and totally fine to need more time for this.

The Three Stages

There are three distinct emotional phases that a new mother will generally go through postpartum. The first is what I call the "taking in." For the first one to three days after you have your baby, you may find yourself just verbalizing, sharing your birth story and going over the finer details. You may still be piecing everything together and recalibrating. You may also find yourself very passive or dependent on others to help you get things done, whether at home or even in the care of your body or baby. Finally, you may experience what I refer to as "blissful surrealism": looking (staring!) at your baby, amazed and even a little dumbfounded.

In the next phase, which will be from roughly day 3 to day 7, you'll build more independence. You'll move through some normal physiological stages of postpartum and begin to understand what your body may be needing. You will also get an idea of the new structure of your days and begin acclimating to that. You may have a stronger interest, and ability to participate, in the care of your baby. All of these things can feel really good. I call this phase the "taking hold."

After about ten days, there's the "letting go." You'll start to understand your new role as a mother (even if only slightly more than before). You'll find yourself in a more active state, learning how you mother. You'll likely feel the importance of your new role; you'll feel the weight of responsibility for your baby as you move into the role of primary care provider. For this reason, you may find yourself shedding any preconceived notions of how you thought you, your baby, or this time was going to or "supposed to" be. Any idyllic notions will start to wash away, replaced by these more real encounters. You also may, for the first time, start to see your baby as separate from you. This can be tough, but it can also be a welcome release; once again, your body is yours and yours alone.

Postpartum Mood Disorders

Even with very little prior knowledge of the postpartum shift, you're probably somewhat aware of the spectrum of mood disorders that can come after birth. These can range from the common yet mild "baby blues" immediately after birth, to postpartum depression, to the rare but extremely serious postpartum psychosis.

Nearly half of all postpartum mood disorders will develop during pregnancy, so pay close attention to how you're feeling during your pregnancy. About 75 percent of women report some type of low, bluesy feelings after delivery, and upward of 20 percent reach a full diagnosis for postpartum depression or anxiety, which means that most—close to all—women experience some level of emotional imbalance at some point in their pregnancy or after they have their baby. In fact, perinatal/postpartum depression is the most common complication of childbirth. If you find yourself thinking, "I just don't feel like myself" shortly after birth, chances are there may be more going on. So let's walk through the characteristics of some of these feelings and become familiar with some of the symptoms; that way you can recognize them if they crop up for you. Remember, they are very normal—and, most important, if you think you may need help, seek it out.

Transition smoothers for each level of postpartum mood disorder follow the descriptions of all three.

The Baby Blues

You may have heard of the baby blues—a common mental and emotional phenomenon that up to 80 percent of women experience after giving birth. It's so common because the pregnancy hormones—estrogen, progesterone, oxytocin—come crashing down to their normal levels after the placenta is delivered. The immediate reduction of hormones after nine months at a higher level can naturally lead to feelings of sadness, irritability, lack of focus, dependency, emptiness, listlessness, and a mild depressive state. It's not uncommon to be weepy, sensitive, or just generally "down" in the first week. It usually lasts for one to two weeks, and it usually disappears as you begin to feel more confident and balanced and your body starts to heal.

Postpartum Depression

Symptoms of baby blues lasting for more than two weeks, or these symptoms appearing two weeks after delivery, are generally considered to be postpartum depression (PPD). Still relatively common, affecting 10 to 20 percent of new mothers, PPD goes beyond baby blues in its intensity and duration. It can take the form of what we typically think of as depression: a generally "gray," muddy feeling; listlessness; crying; lethargy; decreased appetite; lack of interest in taking care of your baby or yourself; and feelings of guilt, shame, or hopelessness. It typically emerges in the first two to three months after birth but may occur at any point within the first two years after delivery.

Postpartum Anxiety

Postpartum anxiety disorders—such as panic disorder, obsessive compulsive disorder, and generalized anxiety disorder—can be as common as postpartum depression and even coincide with general depression. Anxiety symptoms can include the following: panic attacks, hyperventilation, excessive worry, restless sleep, and repeated thoughts or images of frightening things happening to the baby. If you experienced any of this during your pregnancy, it could potentially persist into your early postpartum period.

Postpartum Psychosis

Much like postpartum depression and anxiety, mothers suffering from postpartum psychosis can be anxious, agitated, and suicidal. However, what differentiates a postpartum psychosis case is that the mother will have thoughts of harming both herself and her baby. She may also show signs of cognitive impairment and delusions, and hallucinations. The onset of these symptoms is usually three weeks to three months postpartum. Postpartum psychosis is rare, affecting only about 0.01 percent of new mothers, and clearly must be taken quite seriously. It is considered a psychiatric emergency, and hospitalization will likely be needed.

Transition Smoothers for the Baby Blues

Exercise. The best thing to steady your mind and body as all this newness unfolds has got to be exercise. "Real" exercise—hitting the gym, running, classes, and the like—is not an option before that first checkup with your doctor, but lighter exercise, like walking, is a great idea as soon as you're ready to try it. A long, slow walk in the first week postpartum with your baby will not only help clear your head, but will help your body rehabilitate and regain strength.

Nourishment. Make sure you're eating well and, most important, healthfully.

Meditation. If this book helped you through your pregnancy, you're already well familiar with the Five-Minute Reboot (see page 55 for a refresher). This quick, easy, and refreshing meditation is great postpartum as well, when you may feel like you have only five minutes for yourself. It's also great to do the Five-Minute Reboot if you have trouble napping; take five minutes to follow your breath and look inward, then see if you are able to rest. In pregnancy, there may have been a particular mantra that really resonated with you at a certain time. Revisit it now and see if you find yourself as charged by it.

Rescue Remedy. For acute support with shock, sadness, agitation, loss of control, and feelings of exhaustion, try Dr. Bach's Rescue Remedy, four drops at a time under the tongue or diluted in water.

Bodywork. Get some that first week. Even just a head, shoulders, and foot massage if you had a cesarean birth. A recent study showed that regular massage once or twice per week can lower cortisol (the stress hormone that causes depression and anxiety, as well as high blood pressure and a lower immune system) by up to 53 percent. In the study, about five hundred men, women, and children with depression or anxiety problems all reported feeling their symptoms decrease. Not only does massage decrease cortisol, but it also seems to increase serotonin and dopamine, the two neurotransmitters that help reduce depression.

Transition Smoothers for Postpartum Depression, Anxiety, or Psychosis

Use everything on the baby blues list, and add these:

Talk to your care provider. At times, this could even mean your child's pediatrician. Unfortunately, the system is such that you will not see your OB/GYN or midwife again until the routine six-week visit, unless there is an emergency sooner. Your pediatrician is the best first line of contact because you'll see her often after you have your baby—up to three times in the first month. Let her know any depressive or anxious thoughts you may be having—pediatricians are typically well trained and stay current with research in how to deal with PPD and should be able to give you a good referral to a therapist or psychiatrist. Of course, let your OB/GYN, midwife, or doula know what's going on, and look to them for support.

Have your thyroid checked. Postpartum thyroiditis has many of the same symptoms of some postpartum mood disorders like sadness, moodiness, fatigue, and anxiety. It's estimated that approximately one out of every seventeen women in the United States experience thyroid issues after birth. Pregnancy is a time of complex hormonal changes, so it's a time when women are particularly vulnerable to developing thyroid dysfunction. Once any thyroid issue is treated, usually mood disorders tend to improve quickly.

Explore medication. If a doctor or psychiatrist recommends medication, it may be best to follow their recommendation, even if the idea of medicating yourself makes you hesitate. Most people who go on an antidepressant during pregnancy or postpartum do not need to be on the medication forever. However, studies have shown that there are risks. Women on antidepressants are more likely to give birth prematurely than depressed women who aren't on medication. Other related risks are congenital heart defects, other rare birth defects, clubfoot, and a serious lung condition called persistent pulmonary hypertension. Studies have shown that the risk of certain SSRI medications affecting breastfed babies is extremely low.

Speak to your partner. For whatever reason, in this period of a woman's life many tend to feel that they must be perfect. Letting your partner in and talking about what's going on with you mentally is the best way to find the type of day-to-day support you may need to get you through this time. The sooner you speak up about it and get the help you need—whether it's medication or one of many types of therapy—the sooner you can get back to your life.

Your Birth Story

How did your birth go? Maybe it went just as you imagined—or maybe not. Your thoughts about it may be complicated. You may feel sad, angry, confused. Many mothers feel that birth was worse than they expected; some say they feel traumatized by their experience. Adding to this, your voiced feelings could be met with dismissive attempts to soothe you: "At least you got a healthy baby in the end!" or "But you're fine now!" The truth is, around 30 percent of mothers report feeling at least some-what traumatized by their birth experience, and as many as 9 percent can show symptoms of post-traumatic stress disorder (PTSD) as a result. No matter how big or small this feeling may be, if you're experiencing these types of thoughts, I encourage you to continue to explore them. No feelings are best dealt with through dismissal and denial; try to address these feelings so that you can move forward with your new motherhood (and potential other pregnancies) positively and optimistically.

Here are some transition smoothers for your birth story:

- Journal about it. The best first step for unsettling feelings is always to hit the paper. If it's not too painful, write your birth story and all the details you can remember. Pause at the parts that made you feel poorly and describe what it was about those moments that were upsetting or disappointing.

- Discuss your feelings with someone willing to listen (without dismissing your thoughts). This may be your partner, friends, or someone in your community.

- Revisit the details of your birth with your care provider. If something happened that you were confused by or that felt uncomfortable to you, bring it up with your care provider, who may be able to talk through what happened.

- Reach out to Solace for Mothers, an online support group for mothers traumatized by their birth experience. Speaking to others in your situation can help validate your feelings and help you feel more empowered about your experience.

Your Partner

The nature of your relationship with your partner has likely already changed through your pregnancy. Watching together as your body changes—as your body acts, well, more bodily—can bring on intense bonding as you get especially "real" with one another. Your relationship will continue to shift with the addition of a newborn to your family unit, and navigating that shift can be particularly tricky at times (see page 432 for more on this). You both might find yourselves busy and preoccupied with your baby, thinking less about each other's needs.

Transition Smoothers with Your Partner

- Make time every day to check in with one another—put it in your shared calendar and just make it happen. Express yourself, and don't forget to ask about your partner. Draw out their feelings and take them in without judgment: How is it going? What can I (or can we) be doing better?

- Verbalize the help that you need, and incorporate your partner into the business of baby care. It can be very empowering to feel confidently responsible for a little life; share that with your partner. Don't feel like you have to take on everything yourself.

And If You're Single

- Find your support group—a new mothers group can provide much-needed support. If you don't have a circle readily available, ask your care provider if they know of a group for single mothers. Other trusted loved ones, like friends or even neighbors, can be helpful as well. Even if they themselves are childless, having some extra hands on deck will provide you with the breaks you need.

- Stay positive. Going the road alone will be tough, but it's been done countless times before, and you can definitely do it. Keep your sense of humor about you—laughter is the best medicine and coping mechanism!

Sex and Intimacy

Intimacy can be a real challenge in the postpartum period. While sexual intercourse is not an option in the early days (before your six-week appointment, generally), intimacy is—and certainly should be! Making time to check in with each other and be in touch will naturally remind you that you're a team and that you share a unique bond. From what I've seen, solid verbal communication, as just described, can smoothly and naturally transition into a more physical expression.

While you're breastfeeding, and getting a healthy dose of oxytocin in doing so, your needs for intimacy are somewhat met (albeit differently from partner intimacy), and you might feel less interested in being touched. Your partner will not be enjoying this same hormonal rush and nurturing touch, so it's important to try to draw yourself out of your latency and reconnect. Your interest in penetration may even take a while to return (even after the recommended six-week stalemate); however, approaches like mutual masturbation, oral sex, heavy touching, and making out can certainly help draw you back together.

Here are some transition smoothers for sex and intimacy:

Use lubricant. Your vaginal tissues have stretched and are now contracting, which causes them to be quite tight. Additionally, as you are fairly sated from the release of oxytocin from breastfeeding, you may have difficulty getting as aroused as you may have previously, especially in the early postpartum period.

Take it slow. Not all sex needs to include penetration. You can find other ways to be intimate: deep slow kissing, massages, baths together, or manual stimulation.

Wear a bra. If you're breastfeeding, you might leak during sex. Oxytocin helps your milk let down, but it also helps you orgasm, which could lead to your spraying a little bit on your partner. It happens.

Get prepped. Take 800 mg of ibuprofen thirty minutes before you get busy. It can help minimize the pain from inflammation.

If you continue to have discomfort with sex, get help from a physical therapist who specializes in pelvic floor therapy. These experts can help get you back on track.

....

The 40

This body oil is intended to help uplift, restore, and inspire you as you're making your postpartum shift; think of it as your forty-day ritual in a bottle. Sandalwood is invigorating and provides mental clarity, neroli is an antidepressant, and lavender helps calm and soothe and eases sleeplessness.

¼ cup [60 ml] sweet almond oil

15 drops sandalwood essential oil

5 drops lavender essential oil

5 drops neroli essential oil

Combine the oils in an amber or blue glass bottle with a pump top. Massage the mixture into your skin as needed.

....

YOUR ENVIRONMENT

The people and things we surround ourselves with have an enormous impact, even without the heightened sensitivity and demands that come with pregnancy and postpartum. Now your environment is especially important to help streamline your responsibilities (and burdens) while you acclimate to new motherhood. In the following sections, you'll find advice on everything from where to put a snack station to how much housework you should do (ideally: none).

Nourishment

With exhaustion and other body challenges going on, plus your attention being diverted to your new baby and routine, it can be very difficult to remember to care for yourself, even in the most basic way—by eating nourishing food. Yet food is so important, not only to provide you the energy you need to take on this new phase, early motherhood, but also to help you maintain the milk supply you'll need to, in turn, nourish your baby. Additionally, you will be more sensitive to insulin than you were while pregnant, putting you at risk for severe blood sugar drops. Staying full, grazing throughout the day, will really help. Try and eat every three hours; a great reminder is every time your baby feeds, you should too, right after you're done feeding him. You'll notice that the last two recipes I provided in Chapter Six, Month Nine (pages 163 to 164) are wonderful for making ahead.

Here are a few tips for nourishing yourself in the early months:

- Set up snack and water stations where you'll be nursing and sleeping so you don't even have to think about rehydrating and curbing low blood sugar. Remember, use your baby's feeding as a reminder that you should eat as well.

- Depending on financial parameters, putting some of your budget toward a food delivery service can be a great way to keep your kitchen stocked. Doing this for just one to two weeks in the beginning can take a significant load off of you and your partner. Or if you've had a meal train set up by a friend, look to have something warm delivered every other day. That way you aren't overwhelmed with food.

- For the first few days postpartum, you may actually not feel hungry at all. Don't worry if you're not motivated to eat very much; that's your adrenaline working, which has kicked in to help you with all of the feeding and diaper changing you're doing. Your appetite will return around day 3 or so.

- Swap your prenatal vitamin for supplements that better support your postpartum needs. Consulting a naturopath or integrative medicine doctor might be helpful; they combine conventional Western medicine with alternative or complementary treatments, such as herbal medicine, acupuncture, and stress reduction techniques, all in the effort to treat the whole person. Here are a few supplements that I like to incorporate for my clients after they've discussed them with their care providers:

  * **Probiotic:** Taking one daily helps promote healthy gut function and reduces inflammation. There's a wide range of types, strengths, and brands; if you need some advice on which one is right for you, ask your care provider.

  * **Zinc:** Offers excellent antiviral support and is an overall immune system booster.

* **Vitamin D3:** Supports the immune system and can help with mood improvement.

* **Magnesium:** Helps reset and relax your nervous system and normalize bowel function.

* **DHA (an omega-3 fatty acid):** Boosts energy, brain function, and joint lubrication.

- Hearty, warming, and protein-rich foods (like most of the recipes in our Through the Months sections) are best. This period is not for dieting, especially if you're establishing your milk supply. It's a great time to reach for protein, whole-grain carbohydrates, fiber, and healthy fats. And definitely eat carbs if you're breastfeeding—carbohydrate restriction can negatively affect your milk supply. Dense soups, root vegetable bowls, stir-fries, and a grilled or roasted protein are better, more filling, and more appropriate meals than traditional lettuce-and-tomato salads. Additionally, healthy fats like ghee and coconut oil, fermented foods like kimchi and sauerkraut, and good fiber from foods like brown rice, spinach, kale, and dates will keep your bowels moving along. When you look at your plate, you should always see portions of protein, fat, and fiber. See the charts that follow for examples of some healthy foods to snack on.

Snack Grid

1: Foods high in protein and/or healthy fats

Cheese	Kidney beans	Pesto
Cottage cheese	Pinto beans	Hard-boiled eggs
Yogurt	Chickpeas	Nuts and seeds (almonds, walnuts, sunflower seeds)
Whole milk	Black beans	
Avocado	Edamame	Cured meat or smoked, canned fish (turkey, chicken, roast beef, salmon, tuna)
Nut butters (almond, cashew)	Hummus	

2: Grains

Ryvita (or another whole-grain cracker)	Rice cakes	Whole-grain sourdough or rye bread
Rice paper rolls	Ezekiel and other sprouted grain breads	Corn tortillas
Pita bread	Brown rice	Quinoa

3: Fruits and vegetables

Any combination of prepared vegetables:	Any combination of prepared fruit:	Dried fruits with no added sugar or sulfur:	Any combination of fermented foods:
Celery sticks	Apples	Raisins	Pickles
Carrot sticks	Blueberries	Apricots	Sauerkraut
Pepper slices	Bananas	Dates	Kimchi
Cucumber slices	Melon	Prunes	Tempeh
Cherry tomatoes	Grapes	Goji berries	
Radishes	Cherries	Bananas	
Olives			

>>>

Snack Attack

Consider these simple snack combinations:

- Avocado, cheese, and tomatoes on a rice cake
- Avocado with smoked salmon on sprouted-grain bread
- Cottage cheese with pesto and cherry tomatoes
- Nut butter and banana on toast
- Whole-grain pita with hummus and cheese
- Rice cake with nut butter
- Baby carrots and cucumber slices with hummus
- A cup of steamed edamame with kimchi
- Turkey, cucumber, and cheese in a rice paper roll
- Yogurt with goji berries
- Cottage cheese and blueberries
- Dates stuffed with nut butter
- Pickles and cheese
- Warm milk with cinnamon, honey, and a pinch of sea salt
- Walnuts with dried plantains and cheese
- Pita rolled around a cucumber and cheese
- Turkey and avocado on rice cake
- Apple and celery slices with nut butter
- Hard-boiled egg with cherry tomatoes
- Brown rice with avocado and sauerkraut
- Chickpeas with pesto and cheese
- Black beans, avocado, and cottage cheese in a corn tortilla
- Hard-boiled egg, tuna, olives, radishes, and avocado

Chamomile, Hibiscus, and Lemon Balm Infusion

A natural mixture to cultivate balance, this infusion is rich in nervines (plants that benefit the nervous system), vitamins, and minerals to help soothe and restore your nervous system—a boon for adapting to the needs of your new baby.

Makes 8 cups [2 L]

$1/4$ cup [8 g] dried chamomile flowers
$1/4$ cup [8 g] dried hibiscus flowers
2 tablespoons dried lemon balm leaf

8 cups [2 L] water
1 tablespoon honey or maple syrup

Put the herbs in a mason jar with a lid. Boil the water, pour it into the jar, and allow the infusion to steep for a minimum of 30 minutes and up to 8 hours. Cover tightly with the lid while steeping. After steeping, strain, then stir in the honey and reseal. Keep any leftover infusion refrigerated, and discard after 36 hours.

Buttery Spiced Hot Chocolate

After having a baby, warm fluids are very healing—a perfect reason for a cup of hot chocolate. But this recipe has a twist: It's a little fattier than your usual cup of hot chocolate. Why? Because healthy fat has been shown to provide more energy and help with hormonal balance. The inclusion of grass-fed butter and coconut oil will keep you full, stave off cravings, and provide mental clarity and energy. Plus healthy fats can also help boost your milk supply and the nutrition profile of your milk, if you're breastfeeding. If you want this cup of cacao to act as a meal replacement in the morning, add collagen powder, an easily digestible form of protein that helps with skin, nails, hair, bones, cartilage, and joint repair—all areas in need of support after pregnancy.

Cacao vs Cocoa? *Cacao is chocolate in its most raw form. Packed with magnesium, it can help calm the nervous system and boost the feel-good brain chemical serotonin, which can be in short supply when estrogen levels are at an all-time low shortly after birth. Cocoa powder is more processed, although still a good source of antioxidants and minerals. Therefore, if you can't get cacao, just use cocoa.*

(continued)

Serves 1

1 cup [240 ml] almond milk
1 tablespoon coconut oil
1 tablespoon organic, grass-fed butter
   or ghee
2 tablespoons raw cacao or organic
   unsweetened cocoa powder

1 tablespoon collagen powder,
   preferably Great Lakes brand
1/2 teaspoon cinnamon
1 tablespoon maple syrup or honey
   (optional)

In a small saucepan over medium-low heat, warm the almond milk. Add the coconut oil, butter, cacao, collagen, cinnamon, and maple syrup, if using. Using an immersion blender or a whisk, blend for a minute until frothy. Serve immediately.

Housework

With intermittent periods of bustling activity followed by crashed-out couch sleeping, you may find yourself looking around your home and wondering how everything got so chaotic. Even so: don't do housework, for at least the first week. Right now, this is one of those chores that is best handled by delegation. Ask a close friend, family member, or your partner if they can shoulder it for the next few weeks—or, again depending on financial parameters, this is a great time to budget in some element of housekeeping. If you don't have support, it's helpful to limit your scope—keep one room or one area of the house clean, so that you can go there, away from the rest of the mess, to recharge and gather yourself in a calm environment. This is preferably the place where you're nursing or feeding your baby, so you can relax and drop into that space without any distractions. If you do end up taking on a bit of housework, continue to keep in mind that your abdominal and pelvic organs are still healing; therefore, if you have to work, lie down on your belly for ten to fifteen minutes afterward to help support and soothe your uterus as it heals. Avoid heavy lifting for about two weeks, and never hinge from the waist when bending over. Try to avoiding twisting movements, like sweeping, as well.

Guests and Family

Your community—and in particular certain individuals; you know who they are—can provide either overwhelming support or burdensome stress. You may feel pressure to allow excited family members or friends to visit you at home, or even at the hospital. They can't wait to see the baby and might be quite pushy about it. The same boundaries and personal needs that you established during your birth are in play here. In fact, as a general rule, I recommend giving yourself at least one full week before inviting family and friends over to visit, unless they are willing to roll up their sleeves and pitch in. Think about it: you may not love talking to your partner's sister, but if she's willing to do a pile of dishes you won't really have to! Those individuals are welcome. By two weeks, things won't be perfect, but you'll have a flow going that will make it easier for you to delegate tasks to folks when they stop by, which can feel great for them—most visitors are happy to help. For the more hands-on guests, ask them to read any parenting or infant care books you and your partner love and have decided to adopt; that way they are up to date in terms of philosophy. Times have changed, and updating older family members to your process can be key to consistency (and avoiding tension). If you don't anticipate guests helping (or don't want them to), consult my ideas about hired help in the Getting Help section (page 321).

Once you are ready to let the floodgates open and invite in visitors, be smart about it. Instead of seeing one friend every day, have visit sessions. Pack in a few friends for a visit at a set time—say, between 3:00 P.M. and 6:00 P.M. Then give yourself two days off, with nothing on your calendar, followed by another visit session. Batching visits will help you avoid feeling too exhausted, and following it up with a few empty days will give you a chance to recuperate. Many new mothers complain that the drop-in visitor can be destabilizing. And it can really eat up a lot of your time.

Getting Out

After three days in the hospital or laboring and delivering at home over several days, you may be itching to get out of the house right away. New mothers tend to approach this in many different ways—and you will have your own approach as well. As a general rule of thumb, I recommend waiting two weeks, same as for unwanted visitors. During those first two weeks, your body is undergoing rapid and dedicated healing, which overexerting yourself would only serve to interrupt. Additionally, your baby's immune system is delicate in these early months, but by two weeks she'll be more ready for the outside world (especially with the help of the antibodies in your breast milk, should you choose to breastfeed). You could absolutely try an easygoing walk in a low-impact environment where there aren't a lot of people.

Once you're feeling up for it and your baby is doing fine, ration your various outings. Try not to go out two days in a row—try one day or night out, then two days off, then another day or night out, and so on. This measured spacing will also give you some time to reflect—"Was that OK? Did it feel stressful? How did I feel after being out, and what could I adjust for the next time to feel better?"

The Internet and Social Media

As of publication, we may be safe to assume that this is the only birth and pregnancy book covering Fear of Missing Out (FOMO). I always advise limiting social media intake during early motherhood. The last thing your attention should be wandering toward is, "Oh, I wish I was at that place," or "Wait, all my friends are together and doing what?" The best place for you to be right now is at home, with your baby and your partner—taking care of what's right where you are and keeping what's somewhere else on the perimeter.

If you feel yourself drifting toward social media, try using some of the mindfulness techniques I've laid out in previous chapters (pages 54, 79, 91,

104, 114, 123, 134, 149, and 159). First, take a moment and reflect: Why did you decide to go on your Instagram or Facebook feed? What are you hoping to gain or see? Then: When you go on social media, is there someone in particular you are hoping to catch up on? It may be better to navigate directly to their updates, rather than scrolling through the entire feed. And again: What are your motivations for checking in on that particular person or account? And are they necessary and fulfilling? Try to visit only corners of the social media world that are more restorative and uplifting. If not, save the FOMO for later. Guaranteed, it will be waiting.

In terms of Dr. Google: Avoid. Straight up. If you have pressing questions, reach out to real people and ask for real support. Questions about infant care and your own body are best answered by your pediatrician, OB, or postpartum doula. Having a real, tangible conversation with a qualified person will help you become better informed, and it will also spare you from spinning out with stress from reading dozens of links of questionable advice and downright misinformation.

Getting Help

I really encourage you to seek out and set up some type of at-home help leading up to your delivery. There are many different options, which I'll outline here. Each family has its own financial constraints to consider, and your unmet needs will depend on the degree to which your own family is actually of some help. Take a look at these options and weigh whether any of them feel like a good choice for you.

A family member might offer to come and stay with you, your partner, and the baby to help keep things moving around the house—or help in whatever way you determine. What's crucial about this relationship is that you remain the primary opinion-holder. That means any question about baby care should be directed to you. Always. Depending on your relationship with the family member in question, you may want to postpone accepting their offer to help until after the first two weeks, when you've got a better handle on how you want to do things. It all depends on your relationship and how you jibe with their personality and help style.

A postpartum doula typically comes to your home in the first six to eight weeks—although sometimes for as long as the first six months—to help mother the mother. The primary role of the postpartum doula is to make sure that you as the mother are feeling comfortable and acclimated to your new role. They'll be checking in with you on the progress and sensations of your body, your nutrition, your mental state; they'll also give you objective advice on and support with baby care and, depending on the doula, breast-feeding support. Some even make food.

A night nurse typically works from 10:00 P.M. to 6:00 A.M., and their primary purpose is to help you through the night shift, allowing you to get some much-needed sleep. If your decision is to breastfeed, it's important to speak clearly with your night nurse to establish that and find out how she can help support you in it. She may prefer that you pump (and get up to pump at night) and leave her bottles, or she may bring the baby to you in bed, which is preferable.

Finally, a "mother's helper" is essentially a more hands-on housekeeper. She will come to your house in the daytime and help with everything besides baby care: She might make some food, do some cleaning and laundry, and generally keep the household running smoothly while you focus on tending to your baby.

Keeping It Stocked

You may find that your friends and family are eager to help out but have no clue where to start. A great way that they can truly help is to set up a system for food delivery. There are many different possibilities, depending on your preference. Here are some ideas:

Meal train Someone can set up a meal train for you, or you can set one up for yourself. It's very simple to do on MealTrain.com—choose the time period in which you would like meals delivered, specify any dislikes or dietary restrictions, and email it out to your community or post it on social media. People choose whatever day they're available to drop off a meal. Takethemameal.com is another option that allows you to make a schedule and send a meal too.

Gift cards and credit If cooking seems like a lot of effort—for both you and your community—consider asking for gift cards to your favorite takeout places. Another simple choice is to add Postmates (on-demand delivery) credit to your baby gift registry. (For more registry ideas, consult the Resources, page 431.)

Grocery support Maybe it's not the cooking element that's a challenge, but the shopping. You could tailor your meal train to include biweekly store runs, ask for Instacart (grocery store delivery) credit (if that app services your city), or add membership to a local CSA to your registry. (For more registry ideas, consult the Resources, page 431.)

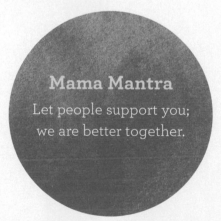

Mama Mantra
Let people support you;
we are better together.

CHAPTER TWELVE

Nourishing and Nurturing Your Baby

You know how, when you're taking a flight, the emergency protocol for a change in cabin pressure is to put on your oxygen mask first before helping others, even children and infants? Well, the last chapter was your mask—in which we looked at meeting your needs—and now that you're up for it, we'll learn how to help your baby.

Providing nourishment and caring for your baby can take a surprising amount of finessing. There's a steep learning curve, but once you've reached the top, I think you'll find that much of the nitty-gritty of mothering starts to come more easily. That said, some things may come surprisingly easily and others be unexpectedly difficult. As I've recommended for each stage of pregnancy and birth, continue to be gentle with yourself in new motherhood, as you discover how to soothe, feed, and simply be with your baby in this new stage of your life. As a golden rule, if you are planning to breastfeed, schedule a visit by a lactation consultant in your home within the first week. Even if things are going well, they can troubleshoot, boost your confidence, and soothe any bubbling anxiety.

BREASTFEEDING

How It Works

At around weeks 16 to 22 of pregnancy, your breasts start to produce colostrum, which will ultimately sustain your baby in the first three days of life. After the delivery of your placenta (either vaginally or surgically if you're having a cesarean birth), your body will rapidly increase milk production and the production of prolactin, the primary hormone that regulates your milk production and supply. When your baby latches on and feeds from your breast, or you pump or hand express, another hormone—oxytocin—is released and causes a milk ejection reflex (MER). Your body responds by contracting the smooth muscles in your breast around the milk ducts that your milk travels through, releasing your milk.

The Stages of Breast Milk

Colostrum (Birth to Seven Days)

This milk is high in protein and low in lactose, and has a laxative effect on your baby to help her make her first poop. It's also rich in antibodies that protect and fortify your baby's gut in this early and vulnerable stage.

Transitional Milk (Seven to Twenty Days)

High in fat and lactose, transitional milk is all about getting your baby to put on weight and poop a bunch—all good things for a newborn.

Mature Milk (Twenty-One Days and Beyond)

Your mature milk contains all of the nutrients and antibodies your baby needs to be nutritionally satisfied and protected. It's a complete meal and all your baby will need for six months, if you decide to breastfeed for that amount of time.

How Long Should You Breastfeed?

There are a lot of opinions and answers to this question! The American Academy of Pediatrics recommends that breastfeeding continue from birth until at least twelve months, and thereafter for as long as you and your baby desire. The World Health Organization recommends continued breastfeeding up to two years of age or beyond. Here's what I think: How long you choose to breastfeed is completely up to you and your baby, and what makes you both comfortable. Sure, we've all heard that breast is best, but your baby will also thrive if formula becomes your best option. Whether it's three days, three weeks, three months, or three years, you and your baby will benefit from breastfeeding.

Benefits of Breastfeeding

Breast milk is perfectly formulated and synergistic with your baby's intestinal system. It's easily digestible and rich in protective enzymes and growth factor hormones; it also possesses antiviral, antibacterial, and antiparasitic properties. It's fascinating—breast milk is dynamic, evolving its makeup and contents along with the age and stage of your baby. The milk you give your baby on day 1 is a totally different mixture than what he drinks on day 10 or day 100.

Breastfed babies enjoy a decreased risk of:

- Ear infections
- Childhood diabetes
- Obesity
- Gastrointestinal and diarrheal infections
- Childhood cancers
- SIDS
- Respiratory infections
- Allergies

Breastfeeding mothers may notice:

- More uterine contractions, minimizing blood loss and encouraging the uterus to tone and shrink back down to its prepregnancy size

- Weight loss

- Increased self-confidence in mothering

- A stronger sense of connection with their baby

The First Forty-Eight Hours

Navigating the realm of new motherhood, it's important to take each moment as it comes—and with breastfeeding, this is especially important. Some of the most challenging obstacles and adversity with breastfeeding happen right at the beginning. These challenges can end your breastfeeding journey before it's even begun. What you do in the first forty-eight hours of your baby's life matters—there's no getting around that. How much stimulation your breasts receive within the first hours after birth can impact your supply months down the line. With that in mind, and before we dive into the finer details of breastfeeding, I'll focus on how to best and most effectively navigate those first forty-eight hours.

Room In

The standard advice you may receive is to take advantage of the hospital staff's support—send your baby to the nursery and get some rest. Of course, your rest is important, but keeping your baby nearby, learning his cues, and being available for on-demand feeding is essential for sustained breastfeeding. If you're in the hospital, ask if it's possible that you and your baby room in together and forgo the nursery. If you're at home, have your baby in a cosleeper or bassinet next to the bed. That way you'll be able to initiate feeding often and can listen for his feeding cues.

Skin to Skin

When you're not nursing and need a break, one of the best places for baby to hang out is on your chest. Being skin to skin has numerous benefits, including regulating your baby's body temperature, heart rate, and glucose levels. Plus, it also helps increase the flow of prolactin and oxytocin in your body, boosting your milk supply while you rest.

Frequency

Your baby was actually not born hungry. In fact, her belly is the size of a shooter marble, with no more than a 2-teaspoon capacity. The aim during this period is to "place a large order" for more milk later on, nursing frequently to stimulate production. Each time you nurse, it boosts your prolactin, which lets your body know to make more milk. Aim to nurse at least every three to four hours or more than ten times in a twenty-four-hour period.

Hand Express

New research shows that hand expression within an hour after birth can help your milk increase earlier and lead to higher milk supply in the next seven to twenty-one days. Before you start a feeding, hand express for thirty seconds to one minute to help encourage the ejection reflex. In between feeds, feel free to hand express every so often—whenever you remember. Aim for at least three times a day. Directions on how to hand express are on page 333. If you're in the hospital, ask for a lactation consultant; or consult your midwife.

Milk Supply

You might be surprised (even alarmed) by how little milk you actually produce in this period. After all, your breasts have probably increased in size considerably. Right now your milk supply is building; expect only a few droplets or spoonfuls if you hand express or pump. And remember: Right now, your baby needs only 1 to 2 teaspoons of colostrum to fill her tiny stomach.

When Breastfeeding Doesn't Go as Planned

It's normal and very common to have trouble establishing breastfeeding—after all, neither you nor your baby has ever done this before. It can take some finessing and some practice. Unfortunately for the mechanics of breastfeeding and the way that women's bodies establish supply, we aren't given much time to negotiate the learning curve. Here are some things you can do to make sure your supply is on the right track, feed your baby the small amount of colostrum she requires right now, and give yourself a bit more of a grace period to establish breastfeeding.

Reach out to a **lactation consultant or counselor** immediately if you haven't had a successful feeding six to twelve hours after delivery, are in pain during the duration of the feed, or have been separated from your baby due to complications—such as your baby's needing to stay in the neonatal intensive care unit (NICU). Ask to be shown how to hand express or pump your breast milk. (Note: Colostrum is very difficult to express with a pump. Hand expression is much more effective during this time, even if you have a hospital-grade double electric pump.)

Hand express at least eight times in the first twenty-four hours, bottling or syringe-feeding expressed milk to your baby until your baby latches on to the breast and feeds successfully.

Keep up the **skin-to-skin contact** as much as possible.

If you and your baby are having trouble establishing a good latch, or you are in pain during feeding, or you're experiencing some other complication that is making feeding tough, there are several different options for helping get your baby colostrum in the first days.

- **Cup or spoon:** Your baby is swaddled and held upright. When the cup is touched to the bottom lip, the baby's tongue will come down and out to lap up the milk. Don't pour it into her mouth; this should be giving her practice to stimulate latching on.

- **Syringe or dropper:** The baby sucks on a finger (yours or a nurse's) while the supplement is slowly delivered by syringe or dropper at the same time.

- **Supplemental nursing system (SNS):** This is a system of tubes that you wear at the breast to entice the baby to feed. This can feel like a complex intervention, but it has proven to be very successful. As the baby breastfeeds, he is able to draw milk from the breast and the SNS at the same time.

- **Nipple shield:** If your baby is having trouble latching, ask your lactation consultant if you may have more success with a nipple shield. A nipple shield is an ultra-thin silicone shield that you place over your breast and nipple that makes it easier for your baby to latch on. Note that using nipple shields at first doesn't necessarily dictate that you'll require them forever. You can use one until your baby's mouth can open wider, your nipples are less sensitive, or you two get into more of a rhythm, then slowly wean your baby off of it. See page 349 for more information.

You've Tried It All, But You Can't Seem to Express Any Colostrum

Take a deep breath. It's OK, go ahead and supplement with formula for a few days. But here's how you protect and boost your milk supply while you supplement.

1. Before each feeding, try and breastfeed first to give you and your baby another chance. If after five minutes the struggles you've been experiencing crop up, offer formula, preferably with you and your baby skin to skin.

2. After offering formula, pump for 15 to 20 minutes and hand express briefly to help stimulate your supply.

3. Repeat these steps at every feeding (so every 3 to 4 hours) until you start to see colostrum when you pump or hand express.

By doing this your baby is getting fed and you are continuing to stimulate your milk supply. It's a win-win.

Ultimate Goals

This is a time of supply establishment and exploration. Stay curious about your body and just observe what's happening. How do your breasts feel, and how do you feel after a successful feeding? You aren't providing your baby with much in the way of nutrition during this time; you should be transferring just enough milk for him to produce at least one wet and one dirty diaper on day 1, and two wet and two dirty diapers on day 2. Try to relax and spend time with your baby on your chest.

Engorgement

For forty-eight hours you've been nursing on demand, rooming in, and snuggling your baby, skin to skin. Then, within three to seven days of delivery, your milk volume will increase. And your breasts may swell—a lot. Engorgement can sometimes lead to pain and sensitivity, and your breasts can get so full that it's very difficult for your baby to even latch on.

Signs of engorgement:

- Fuller breasts (sometimes two sizes bigger than usual) that feel hard or "ropey"; tightly stretched skin that may appear shiny.

- Full ducts that can feel like marble-sized lumps.

- Warmth, tenderness, and/or throbbing that can extend up the breast into the armpit (your armpit has breast tissue too).

- Nipples increased in diameter, becoming flat and taut, making latching on challenging.

- Low-grade fever.

How to find relief:

- Nurse frequently. The best way to work through engorgement is to nurse your baby. Aim to nurse at least eight to twelve times in twenty-four hours.

- Before a feed, use a warm compress to help soften the breast, reduce pain, and help the milk flow. Do not apply a compress for more than five minutes at a time.

- Try reverse pressure softening. Place two fingers on either side of your nipple and press back for fifteen seconds, then release. Move one-quarter of the way around and repeat. This will help press back the fluid buildup and ease pressure on your nipple, making it easier for your baby to latch on.

- Pump or hand express milk before attempting a feeding, just enough to soften the breast for a good latch. Hand expressing is preferred, as breast tissue is more easily damaged during engorgement. If you do pump, aim for a low suction setting and short duration.

- Massage the breast as you feed, using your thumb to stroke from the chest wall all the way to the nipple and moving around your breast clockwise.

- After a feed, use a cold compress of cold cabbage leaves on your breast. Cut off the base of the cabbage, peel the leaves, and leave them in the fridge. Before using, gently crush them in your hands and place directly on your breasts, held in place by your bra. Switch them out every two hours. For a list of my favorite natural cold compresses, see The Goods, page 419.

- If your breasts still feel full after a feed, hand express or pump your breast until you feel relief, generally for two to five minutes. If you do pump when engorged, keep in mind that breast tissue is more easily damaged then, so avoid excessive pumping duration or suction.

Engorgement should not last for more than three to five days; if it does, you should contact your care provider or a lactation professional for support.

The Basics of Breastfeeding

Now that we've addressed both the first forty-eight hours and later concerns like engorgement, let's discuss some of the nuts and bolts of breastfeeding, including the various ways of positioning your baby, understanding hunger cues, and some tools for the most effective pumping.

Hand Expression

This technique can help boost your supply in the first few days; evert your nipple, making it easier for your baby to latch on; and relieve full-feeling breasts in between feeds. Getting the hang of hand expressing takes a little effort; a lactation consultant can show you how (you can also find some good demos on YouTube). If you're trying to express colostrum, use a spoon to collect the drops for your baby. Once your milk increases, you can express into a pump funnel or large bowl.

Method:

Step 1
Gently massage your breasts.

Step 2
Move your fingers on opposite sides of your areola.

Step 3
Press your entire breast back toward your chest.

Step 4
Compress your fingers toward each other, like you're making a sandwich with your breast, moving forward toward the nipple, gliding over the skin, not pulling it. Release the pressure, then relax your hand.

Step 5

Repeat several times. Don't expect anything immediately; it might take up to ten to fifteen compressions before you notice any milk being expressed.

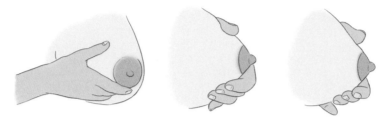

Demonstration of hand expression technique

Massage can help soften breast tissue, which aids in expressing. Do some massage when you feel you may need it or to help you find a full duct. (A full duct might feel like a small pea or a grape.) Massage a full milk duct as you would a sore or tight muscle, using slow, gentle, but firm pressure, releasing as you feel it reduce. A drop or two of massage oil or nipple cream can make this easier.

Positioning and Latch

How you position and latch is unique to you and your baby. What works for you might not work for someone else. What's most important is whatever makes you the most comfortable and allows your baby to feed easily and efficiently. There are several more formalized ways of feeding that you'll be encouraged to try by nurses, lactation consultants, doulas, and the like (we'll discuss those shortly), but if those don't feel like they're working, or you feel uncomfortable or that you're contorting your body, mix it up and try what feels natural. Here we'll explore two different styles of breastfeeding, one that is more traditional and another that is a bit newer. Try both and see how they work for you.

Baby-Led Breastfeeding

Newborn babies may seem like they're not physically capable of much, but in fact, they can really wriggle. New research shows that babies are hard-wired to feed when placed on their tummy on their mother's chest. They can do what's called a "breast crawl": using their primitive newborn reflexes, they can actually move up to the breast and feed with very little assistance from their mother. These reflexes that support the breast crawl persist for at least the first thirty days of your baby's life.

Baby-led breastfeeding (known as "laid-back" or "natural" breastfeeding) takes advantage of these reflexes, and makes for less complicated and more comfortable feeding for you as well. To make a flat enough surface for your baby to wriggle on, you'll need to almost fully recline, which (bonus) takes pressure off of your perineum. It also uses gravity to anchor your baby to your chest and deepen his latch, which is ideal during these early weeks when the baby's mouth is so tiny.

Get a Move On

Your baby's primitive newborn reflexes include:

- Bringing hand to mouth
- Mouth-gaping
- Licking
- Jaw-jerking

- Arm and leg cycling
- Head lifting
- Head bobbing
- Air stepping

Getting into Position

Shift your body. Lean back, using pillows to support your head and arms. You should be in a sloped position, but not flat on your back. You should be able to look into your baby's eyes.

Shift your baby. Scoot your baby onto your chest. Her tummy should be flat against you, with legs in full contact, drawn up like a frog's legs. Make sure your baby's head is higher than her body and that she's near your nipple to allow her to self-latch.

Lift your arms. If your baby moves or rolls slightly, scoot back more to create a more level surface for her, until she's secure when you lift your hands away. Your baby's hands and arms should also be free: This keeps baby calm and allows her to crawl, and her hands can stimulate milk production and milk ejection.

Try different angles. Babies can go to the breast from many angles. Your baby can lie tummy down below your breast either straight or at an angle. After a cesarean birth, try other angles so that your baby doesn't rest on your healing incision.

Shape your breast. Newborns have small mouths, so shaping your breast can help them latch. Place pressure on the top of your breast using two fingers or squeeze the breast, like holding a sandwich, into an oval shape.

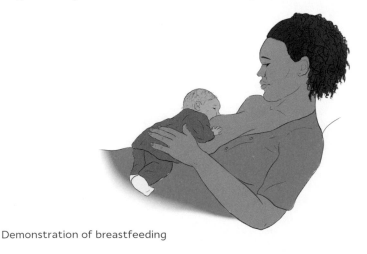

Demonstration of breastfeeding

Quick Reference: Baby-Led Breastfeeding

1. Lean back.
2. Use gravity.
3. Tummy down.

4. Hands free.
5. Self-latch.

Mother-Led Breastfeeding

Baby-led feeding is a relatively new way to approach breastfeeding. The classic style of feeding uses a menu of various positions, postures, and baby-holding techniques to position your baby in a good place to latch. We'll explore these next.

With these techniques, you're in the driver's seat. This may be comforting for you or more in line with how you'd like to parent. Or you may see that your baby is struggling with baby-led feeding and intervene with some of these postures. I wouldn't discount any of these techniques just for being traditional; think of them instead as tried-and-true. Give them a try, experiment with different holds, and always check in with yourself and your baby to gauge what's working.

Things You'll Need for Mother-Led Feeding*

- Nursing pillow(s)
- A small towel or baby blanket
- Footstool

For a list of my favorite products, see The Goods on page 416.

The Method: Cross-Cradle

Place a pillow in your lap and lay your baby sideways, facing you, on top of the pillow. Her ear, shoulder, and hip should rest on the pillow in a straight line, with her tummy facing your tummy. Bring her in close. Use a footstool if your feet don't touch the ground while sitting.

If you're breastfeeding from the right breast, use your left arm to hold your baby, and vice versa.

Make a C-shape with your left hand by spreading your thumb and fore-finger apart. Support your baby's neck in the web between them, wrapping your index and other three fingers behind her neck, cradling her head and allowing it to tilt back a little. Make sure not to press any fingers into the back of her head; this can cause her to arch away from your breast.

With the opposite hand, make a C-shape and gently support your breast, compressing it slightly, as you would if you were holding a sandwich. Make sure the base of your hand is pressed against your chest wall, and keep your fingers off of your areola.

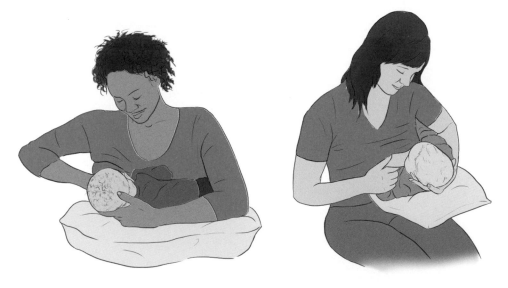

Demonstration of the cross-cradle hold   Demonstration of the football hold

Lift your breast and drag your nipple from your baby's nose to upper lip; this will cue her to open her mouth wide and establish a deep latch. As your baby opens wide, gently push between her shoulder blades with the palm of your hand and bring her in close. Pushing between the shoulder blades will help her head tilt back into the proper position to latch. Never bring breast to baby—always bring baby to breast.

The Method: Football Hold

Place a nursing pillow on the side you'll start from (these steps assume your left breast). Lay your baby on top of the pillow. Her face should be near your breast, with her feet behind your back.

If you need to bring your baby up closer to the breast, tuck a rolled-up baby blanket or towel underneath her head.

Make a C-shape with your left hand by spreading your thumb and forefinger apart. Support your baby's neck in this web, wrapping your fingers behind her neck, cradling her head and allowing it to tilt back a little. Make sure not to press any fingers into the back of her head; this can cause her to arch away from your breast.

With the opposite hand, make a C-shape and gently support your breast, compressing it slightly, like you would if you were holding a sandwich. Make sure the base of your hand is pressed against your chest wall, and keep your fingers off of your areola.

Lift your breast and drag your nipple from your baby's nose to her upper lip; this will cue her to open her mouth wide and establish a deep latch. As your baby opens wide, gently push between her shoulder blades with the palm of your hand and bring her in close. Pushing between the shoulder blades will help her head tilt back into the proper position to latch. Never bring breast to baby—always bring baby to breast.

The Method: Side-Lying

Lie on your side facing your baby with one pillow under your head and one behind your back. Have a rolled-up towel or baby blanket within reach.

Put your baby on his side, facing you, with your nipple in line with his nose.

Bend your top leg, and keep the leg underneath you straight—this will help bring your breast closer to your baby. Rest your bottom hand behind your ear.

Pull his feet and bottom in close to you. Lean back onto the pillow behind you until your nipple lifts off the bed to the level of your baby's mouth.

When your baby opens his mouth wide, press into his shoulder blades with the palm of your free hand to help him latch on deeply (not shown in the illustration). Pushing between the shoulder blades will help his head tilt back into the proper position to latch. Never bring breast to baby—always bring baby to breast.

Wedge the towel or blanket behind his back, leaving his head free to tilt back and rest on the bed.

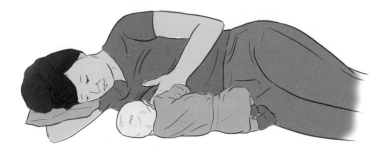

Demonstration of the side-lying position

The Latch-On

You might be hearing a lot of advice about breastfeeding that discusses the latch. If it's done correctly, you and your baby are both happy—you're feeding your baby without pain, and your baby is drinking comfortably from your breast. But what is the latch, and what makes one "perfect"? For most of us, it's been a long time since we were in the driver's seat, drinking milk or formula. We often equate the sucking motion with drinking from a straw, when in fact it's almost the opposite.

A good latch means a deep latch—your nipple will actually stretch and extend to the back of your baby's mouth, spraying milk into her throat. Keep in mind that, unlike the image of a straw, your nipple has between twelve and fifteen openings at the tip. Your baby isn't sucking on your nipple like a straw; she's actually drinking and gulping down the milk. Your nipple stretches to two to three times its resting length when your baby is drinking, extending all the way to your baby's soft palate at the top and back of her mouth. The pain that comes from a poor latch is typically a result of the latch not being deep enough. The nipple ends up pushed against your baby's tongue and/or hard palate.

I encourage you to go with how it feels. If you are in no pain and your baby is drinking well and thriving, you've found your perfect latch, even if it doesn't look like anything you've seen or read.

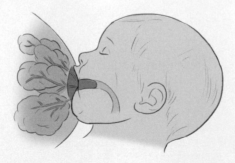

Diagram of proper latch

Burping

Breastfeeding babies drink in a coordinated rhythm that allows them to balance breathing and swallowing, which gives them fewer issues with taking in air. That said, babies do take in some air here and there, which can be very uncomfortable in that little body of theirs. At the very least, it's a good idea to keep your baby upright for five to ten minutes after a feeding to allow him to burp naturally and give him a chance to digest more easily. It can also be a nice time to get a snuggle in as well.

Common signs baby needs a burp:

- Pulling away from the breast during the feed

- Coughing and spluttering at the breast during the feed

- Squirming and grimacing when you lay him down after a feed

If your baby seems to be having trouble getting air out, here are a few methods to try:

The Shoulder Burp Drape your baby way up over your shoulder so that the top ridge of your shoulder presses against her tummy, then rub her back in a fluid and firm upward motion. Hold her securely by hooking your thumb under her armpit. If she's on your right shoulder, hold her with your right hand.

The Chin Burp Seat your baby on your lap and place the heel of your hand against her tummy, with her chin resting on the top of your hand. Lean her forward, resting most of her weight against the heel of your hand to provide counterpressure on her tummy, and pat her on the back to move up the air bubbles.

The Lap Burp Drape your baby over one thigh (legs crossed or spread) so that it presses upward against her tummy. Support baby's head with one hand while you pat or rub her back with the other hand.

The Chest Burp Sometimes babies need help getting air not only out the top end, but also out of the bottom. The knee-chest position (flexing baby's knees up against her chest) helps baby pass excess gas.

If your baby is content, then there's no need to burp. Don't worry if you don't manage to bring up a burp after every feeding, especially after a short or shaky feed. After a longer feed, feel free to put a little effort into burping your baby, but if you don't get a burp after ten minutes, move along.

Feeding Feelings

After pregnancy and birth, you may have thought you were done with new and unusual feelings and sensations. Alas, no: When you're breastfeeding, your body is undergoing a whole new set of physiological adjustments. What follows is a list of some things you may be feeling, which are all totally normal and expected.

Skin sensitivity You might notice that your skin feels tender to the touch, particularly your nipples. Even the feel of clothing might be uncomfortable. That's normal, considering your baby is spending upward of eight hours at your nipple and you haven't experienced that much repeated, extended stimulation in that area. If you can, after each feed leave your breast uncovered to air-dry for a few minutes. Your milk is actually very soothing and hydrating for the area. Even expressing a bit and dabbing it on will be helpful. Hydro-gel pads are also a great help. They're cooling and feel great on the area, plus they offer a buffer between your breast and your clothing, if that's bothering you. Silverettes are small nursing cups made out of 925 silver that help protect the nipples while breastfeeding. Silver is a natural anti-microbial and anti-inflammatory element; it heals and prevents cuts, wounds, cracks, soreness, and infections. These cups can be a great reusable and sustainable alternative to hydrogels.

Fleeting pain When you're first beginning your breastfeeding journey, you may feel pain for the first five to thirty seconds after your baby has latched. The pain should dissipate quickly and get better within the first week. If you're in pain beyond the first thirty seconds of your feed, even on day 1, seek the support of a lactation professional to have a look at your positioning and latch.

Pins and needles You might feel this prickly sensation through your breast and maybe even your armpit (there is breast tissue there, too). This is the milk ejection reflex, caused by your baby nursing. You can experience multiple ejections during a feed, and your baby's crying can cause it as well.

Sleepiness A large amount of oxytocin is secreted during breastfeeding, helping your milk eject and making you feel relaxed and possibly sleepy when a feed is going well. Don't be surprised if you find yourself drifting off during a feed or wanting a nap right after a feed.

Softer breasts Your breasts will feel soft until days 3 to 5, when your milk volume increases. After that your breast will feel full and firm when filled with milk before a feed, and should feel softer after a feed if your baby has fed well. After about three weeks, you might notice that your breasts aren't feeling as full. Don't panic; that doesn't mean there's anything wrong with you milk supply or that it's disappeared. In fact, if your baby is nursing well, breast fullness should last only about two to four weeks. After that the hormones from birth balance out, your milk supply is well established, and your breasts should go back to feeling close to normal.

Your Baby's Cues: Hungry or Satisfied?

Spending so much time with your baby, you'll quickly get a good idea of his various cues. In these quiet early days, it's a great time to just take some pauses and observe your baby. He'll actually be telling you quite a bit about how it's going for him with all those tweaky little movements and deep, restful times as well.

Hungry

Contrary to what you might have previously thought, crying is actually one of the late indications of hunger. Plus, if your baby is crying, it will make it more difficult for her to latch—compounding the problem! If that's the case, try to soothe your baby back to a calm state before attempting to latch. You might be wondering, though: If crying is a late indication of hunger, what's the first or second indication she's hungry? In fact, your baby has three stages of hunger cues: early, mid, and late. Ideally you want to catch your baby between her early and mid cues.

Early Cues	Mid Cues	Late Cues
Waking up	Stretching	Crying
Mouth opening	Stirring	Turning red
Turning the head, seeking and rooting	Tongue thrusting	
	Bringing hands to mouth	

Satisfied

In these early days, the clearest sign that your baby is sated will probably be when he's calmly and serenely asleep. These moments will bring you pride—you're feeding your baby! There are, of course, a number of other indications that your baby is feeding well. Prepare to swell with pride over a floppy baby and wet diapers. It happens to the best of us.

Visible sucking and audible swallowing When your baby latches, there will be a short, fast burst of sucking visible at the cheeks as your baby stimulates the milk ejection reflex. Once the milk has come down, the suck pattern should weaken, slow down, and be interrupted by gulps. If the room is quiet, you should be able to make out a faint "pah-pah" or "kah-kah" as baby swallows gulps of milk. Your baby will swallow after every one or two sucks.

The Flop When your baby is hungry, you'll notice lots of tightness in her hands and body. After a feed her body should be relaxed, so much so that when you lift her hand up it should be unfurled and flop right back down against her body. Her suck will also become weaker and less consistent.

Wet and dirty diapers This is the best way for you to tell if your feedings are going well, because full tummies lead to lots of full diapers. Expect one wet diaper and one stool on day 1, and up to six to eight wet diapers and three stools per day by day 6 of life. Also look at the stool color. If breastfeeding is going well, your baby's stool will turn from black to green by about day 3 and green to yellow by day 4 or 5. If you're seeing fewer diapers than that, it could be a sign that your baby is not drinking well from the breast and you should seek lactation support.

Weight gain This is another concrete way to tell whether or not your baby is feeding well. Babies normally lose about 5 to 7 percent of their birth weight during the first three or four days. Your baby should begin gaining weight around day 5, and should regain or exceed his birth weight by day 10 to 14. If your baby is not putting on weight at this rate, it could be a sign that your baby is not drinking from the breast well.

Sleep Well-fed babies tend to sleep after feeding. After a good feed, expect at least one to three hours of shut-eye. If your baby is struggling to stay asleep for more than ten minutes, this could be a sign that he is still hungry or not feeding well at the breast.

How Often?

Aim to breastfeed every three to four hours and your baby should be feeding ten times or more in a twenty-four-hour period. As adults we tend to find comfort in clear guidelines and straightforward scheduling. Your baby is not like that. In fact, scheduling your baby's feeds is counterintuitive to how your baby is processing the world right now—she has no concept of time. She may feed every fifteen minutes for two hours and then sleep for four. She may be on a regular feeding routine, every two hours, then drop into a deep, restorative sleep to help her grow and develop. For this reason, it's best to nurse on demand, following the cues just outlined. Remember that as long as your baby fits in about ten feedings a day, is producing lots of wet and dirty diapers, and is gaining weight, it's working perfectly.

And How Long?

The length of your feed and whether you offer your baby one side or both breasts is completely unique to you and your baby. Again: If your baby is showing all the signs of feeding well, there's no need to change anything; you've hit the perfect length. That said, there are a few starter guidelines that can be helpful for new breastfeeding mothers. Start with these and then alter them for your and your baby's routine.

The minimum and the cozy maximum Breastfeed for a minimum of ten minutes and a maximum of as long as you like. I like to say thirty minutes on each side is a cozy maximum, but that's really up to you and your baby. (Try not to compare how long your baby feeds to how long another baby feeds. Every baby eats at his own pace; there are fast eaters and slow eaters.) A good way to know that your baby is done feeding is to look for a change in his suck: At the beginning, his suck will be strong and frequent. This is called "nutritive sucking." When he starts to become full, his suck will become less strong and less frequent, called "nonnutritive sucking." His body will be more relaxed then—check for the flop.

One breast or both? If your preference is to offer both breasts per feed, keep in mind that your baby will more than likely feed longer on the first breast. Think of it as main course followed by dessert. If you find your baby getting sleepy in between breasts, burp and change her before offering the other side. If you're offering one breast per feed, make sure to alternate each breast equally within a twenty-four-hour period so that the milk supply is the same for each breast.

Your supply and baby's capacity Many women say that their biggest breastfeeding worry is not having enough milk for their baby. Let me put your mind at ease. Most women will make enough milk to feed their baby; this misconception comes from growing up seeing pictures of babies drinking big bottles of milk and thinking that when your baby is born you'll need to have buckets of milk ready and waiting. As I've stressed, at birth your baby's tummy has a very limited capacity, and your milk supply matches that. Don't forget, your breasts start to produce milk around weeks 16 to 22 of pregnancy.

Your Baby's Tummy Size

- **Day 1**—Size of a cherry / 1 to 1½ teaspoons
- **Day 3**—Size of a walnut / 0.75 to 1 ounce [20 to 30 g]
- **Day 7**—Size of an apricot / 1 to 2 ounces [30 to 55 g]
- **Day 14**—Size of an egg / 2 to 5 ounces [55 to 140 g]

A Few Common Breastfeeding Challenges

Flat or inverted nipples Flat or inverted nipples can make feeding more challenging and potentially painful. To check if you have flat or inverted nipples, try the following: Place your thumb and index finger above and below your areola, and gently squeeze your two fingers together. A typical nipple will stick out when squeezed; a flat nipple flattens or moves inward, retracting toward your chest wall when squeezed; an inverted nipple tucks into the areola when squeezed. If you have flat or inverted nipples, make sure a lactation consultant comes to see you within twenty-four hours after you've delivered. Your baby's sucking on your nipple might help resolve the issue, and it might evert on its own; however, it may be best to use nipple shields to help make feeding easier until that happens. TheraShells, made by Medela, can be helpful to wear in between feeds; they can help both evert the nipple and protect it from coming into contact with clothing. Silverette is another sustainable option.

Nipple pain Continuous nipple pain is usually related to poor positioning or a poor latch. Take a look at the sidebar on deep latching (page 341) and seek out advice from a lactation professional if pain persists. If, after that's been corrected, you're still experiencing unexplained pain, ask your pediatrician if your baby may have tongue-tie—a short band of tissue between the tongue and the floor of the mouth. Babies with tongue-tie can overcompensate by sucking very hard, which can cause nipple pain and even damage.

Too little or too much milk In most cases, the amount of milk your baby extracts from the breast will dictate the amount of milk your breasts produce; supply matches demand. That said, some women do under- or overproduce, which can be difficult and disheartening. If you're concerned that your baby isn't getting enough milk or that it's difficult for your baby to feed because you have too much milk, consult the sidebar Half Full or Half Empty? for self-diagnosis and some easy things you can do to adjust your supply. If the problem persists, consult your pediatrician or lactation consultant for assistance.

Plugged ducts Milk flows through a duct system in your breasts. Sometimes parts of the ducts can become blocked, which causes the milk flow to get backed up. A plugged duct can happen if your baby is not latching or draining your breast well, or if you've gone too long between feeds (more than six to eight hours). If you have a plugged duct, you might feel a hard lump near the plugged duct. It may feel tender, hot, or swollen or look reddened. Your breast might be unusually tender and painful in a certain section. If the blockage is not treated, the area may become infected.

Mastitis An untreated plugged duct can become mastitis if not treated. Mastitis can also be caused by bacteria entering the breast. It usually occurs within the first three months of breastfeeding. Unlike a plugged duct, you'll have more symptoms, like breast pain, swelling, warmth, fever, and chills. Mastitis can be treated with antibiotics, but there are alternative treatments. It's a common myth that it is unhealthy for your baby to breastfeed while you have mastitis. This is false; the antibacterial properties of breast milk protect the baby from infection.

Half Full or Half Empty?

Indications of low milk supply:

- Not enough wet and dirty diapers (there should be six or more wet diapers per day by day 4). If your baby is meeting that output, then you do not have low milk supply.

- Slow weight gain.

- Crying at the breast while latched.

- Not sleeping for more than thirty minutes at a time.

If you think you have low milk supply:

- Contact a lactation professional and set up an in-person visit.

- Drink liquids only to satisfy your thirst (don't force liquids—drinking extra water does not increase supply).

- Make sure you're eating enough protein, fat, and complex carbohydrates and taking in enough calories.

- Pump for five to ten minutes after every feed for twenty-four hours and see if there is any improvement in your supply.

- Get skin-to-skin contact in bed and nurse with your baby for a full day (called a nursing vacation).

- Consider a galactagogue (lactation promoter), like Motherlove's More Milk Plus. You can also turn the Nettle Raspberry Infusion (recipe on page 98) into a lactation-promoting tea by adding 2 tablespoons fennel seeds.

Indications of oversupply or a fast milk ejection reflex (MER):

- Gulping, gasping, coughing, gagging, choking sounds as though the milk is coming too fast.

- Pulling off the breast often while nursing.

- Clamping down on the nipple as if to slow the flow of milk.

>>>

- Making a clicking sound when nursing.

- Spitting up very often and/or tending to be very gassy.

- Periodically refusing to nurse.

If you think you have an oversupply or a fast MER:

- Try baby-led nursing and lean back when you feed. Gravity can help slow the flow of milk.

- Once baby is latched, press gently on your areola using your index and middle finger. This scissor-hand pose can help slow the flow from your milk ducts. Try this for the first two to five minutes of the feed, taking breaks as needed to avoid getting a cramp in your hand.

- Try the side-lying position, which allows your baby to dribble extra milk out of her mouth if it's coming too fast. Make sure to lay down a towel underneath ahead of time.

- Offer one breast per feeding. If your baby finishes nursing on the first side and wants to continue breastfeeding within a two-hour period, just put him back onto the side he just finished off on. This is called block feeding and can help deal with flow issues and help regulate your supply.

- Burp your baby frequently while feeding, taking at least one to three breaks.

Quick Tips for Treating
a Plugged Duct or Mastitis

- Nurse frequently and empty the breasts thoroughly. Aim to nurse at least every two hours. Keep the affected breast as empty as possible, but don't neglect the other breast.

- When unable to breastfeed, express milk frequently and thoroughly (with a breast pump or by hand).

- Use heat and gentle massage before nursing.

- Massage and compress the breast while feeding to help remove the milk.

- Contact a lactation professional or pediatrician for a treatment plan.

A sleepy baby This sounds adorable, I know, but it can be frustrating when your baby falls asleep whenever you bring him to the breast—and then he isn't gaining weight. Some babies are excessively sleepy in the first few days of life. In this case, you might find it helpful to actually wake your baby to nurse on a more rigid schedule—say, every three hours. If he falls asleep while feeding, massage your breast as you feed. This will help eject more milk and keep your baby interested. Once your baby has established a good weight gain pattern, or is having the right number of wet and soiled diapers, it's not necessary to wake him to feed—he will rouse himself. If you are waking your baby for feedings, there are a few techniques that are helpful to rouse him: skin-to-skin contact can be helpful, as can running your nipple across his mouth, holding him in a more upright position, or changing his diaper before the feeding.

Growth spurts and cluster-feeding Expect your baby to be voraciously hungry around the two-week and four-week mark—followed by a significant amount of growth (time to debut the next size up of baby clothes!). When cluster-feeding, your baby may need to nurse every one or two hours, or even continually for several hours. Growth spurts typically last for about twenty-four to forty-eight hours, so although it can feel exhausting, know that you and your baby should cycle back to a more predictable feeding routine very soon.

Alcohol You might find yourself itching for a glass of wine or a cocktail now that baby is here—and you deserve it! But you might also be wondering if it's all right for your baby. Less than 2 percent of the alcohol consumed by you reaches her blood and milk. Alcohol peaks in your blood and milk approximately one-half to one hour after drinking. Alcohol does not accumulate in breast milk; it leaves the milk as it leaves the blood. There shouldn't be a real need to "pump and dump." A perfect time to have a glass of wine would be in between feeds. When your blood alcohol levels are back down, so are your milk alcohol levels. That said, if you're too drunk to drive, you're too drunk to breastfeed. If that is the case, then make sure to pump. You can choose to dump that milk or you can freeze it, label it as boozy milk, and offer it to your baby when she is older than three months. Newborns have very immature livers, so minute amounts of alcohol can tax their system up until three months of age; beyond that they can metabolize alcohol at a faster rate.

Marijuana The American Academy of Pediatrics states that marijuana should not be used while breastfeeding. The long-term effects of marijuana exposure through breast milk are unknown. The active ingredient in marijuana, THC, will be stored in your fat tissues for long periods (weeks to months) and will build up in the body with continued use. Your baby's brain and body are made with a lot of fat; therefore, since your baby's brain and body may store THC for a long time, it's best to pass on that puff or the special brownies or tinctures.

Extra help Professional lactation support can be crucial to your long-term breastfeeding success. Book an in-home visit within the first three to five days after you get home. Visits at home can help quickly correct any critical issues you might be experiencing or provide a simple confidence boost if all is well. In-home visits work well because your provider can see how you and your baby are nursing in your natural environment and quickly make improvements based on how you operate at home. A lactation visit in their office can also be very helpful, but sometimes it can be hard to replicate what you've learned in the office once you get home, so make that a follow-up visit. Online and IRL support groups can also be really great—check La Leche League or KellyMom online; ask your pediatrician for recommendations for local drop-in support (baby gear boutiques can be a good resource).

PUMPING

Using a breast pump can help you gather colostrum in the early days, introduce a bottle, or stockpile milk if you're heading back to work within a few weeks. Pumps are a helpful tool, but it's important to keep in mind that a pump is a less sophisticated method of milk removal—your baby does a better job getting the milk out. Don't worry if not much milk comes out the first few times you use a pump. This is normal; it can take a few pumping sessions for your breast and body to acclimate to the pump. Over time, you'll express higher volumes. Patience and comfort are key factors on your pumping journey. In the following sections, we'll address some of the common questions about how to start pumping, the various types of pumps, and some tips for pumping success.

When to Get Help

Call a lactation consultant or pediatrician immediately if your baby has:

- A day with no wet diapers or bowel movements

- Dark-colored urine after day 3 (should be pale yellow to clear)

- Dark-colored stools after day 4 (should be mustard yellow, with no meconium)

- Fewer wet diapers and stools, or nurses less frequently, than the goals listed in the Satisfied section (page 346)

Or if you have:

- Plugged ducts

- Mastitis

When to Start, When to Pump, and How Long to Pump

Pumping is definitely a foreign concept for new mothers, and all the little intricacies can make it a bit daunting to start. Let's address some of the first, basic questions that might come to mind to get you and your pumping practice up and running.

When to start In general and if all is going well, two to three weeks postpartum is a great time to introduce a pump (especially if you're preparing to return to work). Of course, there are other factors that could get you pumping earlier: baby isn't latching well, you're experiencing mastitis, or if you need to relieve engorgement. Aside from those, it's best to wait until you and your baby establish both your milk supply and a daily feeding rhythm.

When to pump Pumping one to two times per day should suffice to get a nice stock of milk for your baby. I like to advise new mothers to pump in the morning after the first feed and then again right before going to bed. That said, listen to your body and see what time works best for you. Maybe the best time of day for you to pump is in the evening.

How long to pump Aim to pump for at least ten minutes, but no more than twenty minutes. Ten minutes is enough time to stimulate the milk ejection reflex; more than twenty minutes can be overstimulating for the breast (unless directed otherwise by your care provider). If you are exclusively pumping, which means not breastfeeding at all and feeding your baby only expressed milk, you will need to pump much more often than twice a day. The first week after delivery, you should pump at least eight to twelve times per day, along with frequent hand expression sessions. At the two-week mark, your milk supply should be established and you can switch to pumping around seven times per day with the goal of yielding at least twenty-four ounces total per day. If you choose to pump exclusively, work closely with a lactation professional to create a custom plan.

Types of Pumps

There are three types of pumps available for new mothers these days—hospital grade, personal pumps, and hand pumps. Which type you go for will depend on your needs. Will you be taking it with you to an office? Will you be expressing away from home, or is it mostly for home use? If you don't really know yet, that's fine: in the meantime, you can actually rent hospital grade pumps (the breast shield and tubing will be your own) to help you get established.

Another thing to note about pumps: You may be able to work with your insurance provider to cover the cost of the pump. In some cases, they may dictate which pumps they cover. This will certainly make the decision easier for you (by making it for you!), but in my experience, most insurers will cover some really great pumps. Definitely worth looking into.

Hospital Grade Pumps

There are two main things that distinguish a hospital grade pump from a normal, personal pump: Typically the motor is stronger, and it's packaged in such a way that there isn't cross-contamination between users (it also makes the thing much, much bulkier). Because of a stronger motor—and therefore suction—these are the best option if your baby is struggling to latch after delivery or if you're having early breastfeeding trouble.

Personal Pumps

These pumps are similar to the hospital grade ones, but are smaller, lighter, and typically very portable. Some even have battery operation or car chargers, so you wouldn't even need to plug into a wall outlet to use them away from home. These are the most common pumps used and are great for mothers returning to work or traveling, or who just require some degree of flexibility. Because of the structure of these pumps, they cannot be shared between women.

What to Look for in a Pump

Warranty Choose a pump with a least a one-year warranty on the motor.

Fit Your nipple will elongate and change in size as you pump. Make sure that the pump you choose comes with various sizes of breast shields so you can find the best fit (more on that shortly).

Suction and speed The more adjustable your pump suction and speed are, the easier it'll be for you to customize and find your unique settings. Look for a pump with at least two adjustable knobs.

Power Choose a pump that can be run by batteries, a car adapter, and an AC adapter.

Cleaning Check how many parts need to be washed and whether the hard-to-clean tubing ever needs to be cleaned.

Hand Pumps

Also called manual pumps, these are very simple mechanical devices. You simply squeeze a handle, which creates suction and expresses the breast milk. Since you'll be hands-on when using a hand pump, you can express only one breast at a time, which is proven to yield less breast milk. Yet they're a good choice if you're planning to pump only once per day or are looking for a simpler, more lo-fi experience. They can take some getting used to, but many mothers do get through that learning curve and end up loving this option. Also, hand pumps are fairly inexpensive, so it's a good idea to have one and be familiar with how it works in case of a power outage or as a general plan B.

Breast Shields: A Primer for the Best Fit

The fit of your breast shields is key to your pumping comfort. The breast shields are the part of the breast pump that is held against your breast and funnels the milk while you pump. Your breast size doesn't determine the size of your breast shield; rather, it's the diameter and size of your nipple. A comfortable fit means that your nipple moves freely in and out of the tunnel of the breast shield while pumping. If the fit feels tight and there is pain while pumping, choose a larger shield; if the shield is too large, so it doesn't have an airtight seal and some of your breast tissue is drawn into the shield when you pump, choose a smaller shield. Most pump manufacturers make multiple pump sizes. (See the Resources, page 416, for recommendations.)

Making the Most of Your Pumping Experience

Start strong. Turn the pump up to the highest speed setting you can handle without any pain or discomfort until your milk releases. Once it releases, you can slowly start to lower the speed slightly. If you start on a lower speed setting, it will more than likely not be enough suction or speed to trigger the milk ejection reflex, resulting in a longer and less efficient pumping session.

Two-phase expression electric pumps have a mechanism that creates this dynamic without your having to do it yourself. The suction speed is fast for the first two minutes, stimulating the breast; this stimulation phase runs for the average time it takes for a milk release. It then shifts to a slower speed and longer draw, which is how your baby suckles at the breast after milk is released—this is called the letdown phase. This can be helpful, but if you find that you haven't had a milk release by the time the second phase kicks in, you can always press the stimulation phase button until your milk ejects.

Lube up. Place a pea-size amount of nipple cream on your nipple before putting on your breast shield. This will make the suction on your nipple more comfortable as it moves through the tubing.

Get hands free. Use a hands-free pumping bra. These simple bras have holes cut for the breast shields so that you can pump without having to hold them in place. This frees your hands so you can massage and compress your breasts while pumping, or grab a glass of water or a quick snack.

Get hands on. Using your hands to massage and compress your breasts while you pump can help boost your yield by up to 48 percent, and studies show that it can increase the amount of fat-rich and calorie-dense milk you express. Make a C-shape with both your hands by spreading your thumb and forefinger apart. Place both your hands over the breast shields and your breasts, and gently massage in a circular motion, holding the breast shields firmly in place to maintain the suction. Concentrate on the areas of your breasts that feel full. Do this every few minutes while you pump.

Warm up. Using a warm compress on your breasts during pumping is shown to improve your yield by up to 40 percent. In between massaging or while you massage, you can also gently press a warm compress around the exposed areas of the breast in a clockwise direction.

Get distracted. If your hands are free while you pump, divert your attention. Focusing on your breasts and how much is coming out can inhibit your milk ejection reflex. It's best to relax: Watching something on TV or listening to a podcast, or even covering your breast with a shawl might really help your mind relax and let your body do the work.

Add some lavender. Lavender essential oil helps promote relaxation and can be used on the skin. Place one or two drops on your chest (not on your breasts) and rub it in gently; right before you start to pump, inhale deeply. Relaxation can help promote more milk release, increasing your yield.

Milk Storage and Best Practices

Now that you're a pumping pro, you'll need to store all that pumped breast milk! Here are some quick best practices on storage and food safety.

How Long to Store Milk

Your milk can stay . . .

. . . at room temperature for six to eight hours.

. . . in the refrigerator for five to eight days.

. . . in the freezer for two to six months.

. . . in a deep freeze for six to twelve months.

Bottles or Bags?

The choice is up to you and should be based on convenience. A recent study showed that glass bottles and plastic bottles led to less fat loss in stored milk, and it was easier to swirl and reconstitute the milk in bottles than in bags, because the fat in the milk can stick to the bag and be difficult to incorporate. That said, bags are easier to store and can be very convenient, especially if you're on the go.

>>>

Thawing and Warming Breast Milk

- Defrost the milk in the refrigerator overnight (the ideal way, if you can remember).

- Use a bottle warmer, which heats the milk to an appropriate temperature for breast milk. Alternatively, hold the container under warm running water for a few minutes, or submerge the container in a bowl of warm water (just make sure none of the water can seep into the bottle or bag).

- Gently swirl the milk to incorporate the fat deposits that may have separated.

- Use thawed milk within twenty-four hours.

- Never shake the milk, as that can damage the molecular structure that is vital to your baby.

- Never microwave the milk.

- Never heat the milk on a stove burner.

FORMULA AND OTHER BREAST MILK ALTERNATIVES

Breastfeeding may be the biological norm, but there are women who forgo it, for a variety of reasons. It may not feel like the right fit for you; it may conjure past trauma; you may have a medical complication preventing successful feeding; you may have supply issues, inverted nipples, or other breastfeeding struggles. Whatever your reasons, you will know whether and when to opt for formula instead of breastfeeding. The switch to formula can be emotional and difficult for many new mothers—it's another time when things may not be going as you had hoped and planned. You may have to adapt; you may have to find confidence in your decisions from within. If you find yourself dealing with these types of feelings, I advise you to step back to Chapter Seven for a refresher on confidently doing what's right for you and what's right for your baby. Only you can know and make that decision.

Now let's look at the different formula options—and some other feeding alternatives you may not have considered.

Formula

There are three types of formula available: powdered, liquid concentrate, and ready-to-feed. Choosing a formula will depend on how much you'll need, your budget, and advice from your pediatrician. For example, if you're using formula to supplement breastfeeding, you may not need as much and might feel that a pricier option would work well. As always, it's all about what works for your baby. If your baby is under a month old, go with the formula recommended by your pediatrician, which will likely be ready-to-feed because powdered formula isn't sterile, making it potentially taxing to young immune systems.

Powder In a canister with a little scoop, this is the most economical formula on the market. When you're out and about with baby, you'll need to take along water to mix with the powdered formula.

Liquid concentrate This type is more expensive than powdered formula, but it's less messy to prepare. It's a concentrate, so you'll need to add some water to make it drinkable before you give it to your baby. Take along a water bottle if you're going to be out and about.

Ready-to-feed You don't need to add any water to this before feeding—it's perfectly constituted. But if you're on a budget, you'll probably want to go a different route. Of the three formula preparations, ready-to-use is the most expensive.

Alternatives to Formula

Human donor milk This is expressed breast milk sold or donated to a human milk bank. Human milk banks have strict screening procedures, including blood testing. Milk that comes from a human milk bank is pasteurized, so it's safe for another baby to drink (although pasteurization deactivates some vital nutritional properties of the milk). That said, it is a superior option to formula if your baby is premature or has a compromised immune system. The Human Milk Banking Association of North America interviews and

Choosing a Formula:
The Dos and Don'ts

- Follow the formula preparation directions closely.

- Do choose organic and non-GMO. These manufacturing processes are mandated to source their ingredients from farmers who do not use genetic engineering or ionizing radiation in their growing practices. The cows must be fed organic feed, and raised with direct access to the outdoors and without the use of antibiotics or growth hormones. The farms themselves must also pass an inspection by a federal certifier, who makes sure these guidelines have been followed.

- Do choose dairy. Soy is a rich source of plant-based estrogen, which can mimic sex hormones in the body. It's not an issue for older children or adults, but for babies under six months it's best to avoid it. Cow's or goat's milk is a better choice.

- Do use filtered water and invest in a good carbon filter. If that's not possible, use distilled bottled water. Three-gallon water containers with a spout at the bottom are an easy way to use purified water for your baby.

- Do let your baby decide. It all comes down to which formula works better in your baby's tummy. If he gets uncomfortable or gassy or has any other digestive trouble, try a different formula.

- Do check the expiration date on the formula container; make sure it is not damaged, and write down the lot number in case of recalls.

- Do focus on cleanliness. Wash your hands thoroughly before preparing formula. When you open the container, check for foreign particles (insects and pieces of glass have caused some past recalls) or, in liquids, curdling or discoloration.

- Do mix and measure carefully. For powdered formula, use filtered or distilled water; pour it into a clean baby bottle and add the specified measure of formula.

- Don't warm the bottle in a microwave. This can create hot spots in the milk that could be too hot for your baby's mouth. Use a bowl of hot water or a bottle warmer.

- Do store your mixed formula in the back of the refrigerator, where it is coldest.

- Do discard any unused prepared formula after twenty-four hours in the fridge.

- Don't ever freeze formula.

- Do use a cooler with ice packs to transport bottles.

- Don't use formula that has been at room temperature for more than two hours. If your baby doesn't finish a bottle, discard the leftovers.

vets donors based on their health and lifestyle, and screens milk for bacteria before processing, pasteurizing, and bottling it. Casual milk sharing between acquaintances, friends, and family can be risky and is not recommended by the American Academy of Pediatrics, due to risks of infection.

Homemade formula If you're up for it, you can also make your own formula for your baby. This formula is appropriate only for babies over a month old. Look for bulk ingredients to cut the cost. Many mothers like this option because they have direct control of the ingredients they're feeding their baby. That said, it can be quite a commitment. It's clearly the most labor-intensive option available, but it can be done. Take stock of your time limitations and definitely do some research to decide if this is the right option for your family. You can check out the Weston A. Price Foundation for more on making your own infant formula (www.westonaprice.org/beginner-videos/baby-formula-video-by-sarah-pope-2).

Choosing a Bottle

Shopping for your new baby is pretty fun, but it can also be overwhelming due to the sheer amount of stuff available—every one of which claims to be the best. Bottles are squarely in the overwhelming category. Here, let's look at some of the features to look for; as always, take a look at The Goods (page 414), where you can find my recommendations. All of the bottles listed there meet the following criteria:

The nipple When choosing a nipple, take into account the length and the base (the lower part of the nipple, like the areola of your breast). The length should mirror how far your nipple reaches into your baby's mouth, keeping in mind that the human nipple stretches two to three time its normal length when a baby is suckling. You can help re-create this by choosing a bottle nipple with a length that is longer than the resting length of your nipple. As for the nipple base, your baby should be able to accept the nipple and a portion of the nipple base, just as their lips would rest on the areola if you were breast-feeding. This will help encourage a wide and deep latch versus a pinched latch, making the transition between breast and bottle easier.

The flow Also called the flow rate, this term refers to how fast the milk comes out of the nipple. Flow is an integral part of bottle feeding success. If the nipple flow is too fast, your baby might splutter and fuss as she tries to drink, but if it's too slow she might gag and cry as she struggles to extract the milk. Err on the side of a slower flow, increasing as your baby grows.

The texture Nipples that are on the harder side can cause your baby's mouth to tire quickly. If too soft, the nipple can collapse under the pressure of your baby's sucking, causing his lips to roll inward and leading to a pinched latch and possible pooling of milk in the sides of his mouth. Choose a soft to firm silicone-based nipple that has enough give and resistance to stand up to your baby's strong compression when he sucks.

Pace Feeding

Contrary to how you may have fed a baby doll as a kid, the best method isn't to hold a bottle vertically to feed a fully reclined baby. In this position, your baby has no control over how much or little she eats. Pace feeding is a technique more like breastfeeding, which allows baby to regulate her own intake. Here are some tips for pace feeding.

- Feed your baby only when she is showing signs of hunger (see Your Baby's Cues, page 345, for a refresher). This will help you avoid overfeeding.

- Hold your baby semi-upright or upright. Tap her lips with the nipple or gently drag the nipple from her nose to her upper lip until she opens wide. Never force the nipple into her mouth.

- Help your baby latch far enough onto the nipple. Her lips should close on the nipple's base rather than around the tip. If her lips are pulled in, use your fingers to flange them out, but also consider getting a softer nipple that encourages her lips to flange on their own.

- Hold the bottle at a slight angle, so the flow isn't too fast.

- Take a break every few minutes by tilting the end of the bottle so milk runs out of the nipple back into the bottle. Attempt to burp your baby during this break. Two to three breaks per bottle is ideal.

- Repeat throughout the feed until baby is full. Stop when baby stops, even if there's milk left in the bottle; there is no need to force him to finish it.

- If you start feeding your baby on his left side, halfway through the feed switch sides and feed him on his right side. This simple move promotes visual stimulation and development of eye muscle strength.

- Make sure to burp your baby after feeding, to bring up any swallowed air.

Hello, Yellow: A Note about Jaundice

Jaundice is a common newborn condition that usually appears on the second or third day of life. Approximately 60 percent of babies experience some form of it. Jaundice presents first as yellowness in baby's face and eyes, then the chest and stomach, and finally, the legs. The yellow coloring is caused by an overproduction of bilirubin, a by-product of the normal breakdown of red blood cells. Most babies get jaundice because their livers are inefficient during the first few days of life and their bodies create excess bilirubin faster than their livers can break it down and poop it out. Other signs include lethargy and fever. Call your pediatrician if you think your baby might have jaundice.

The most common types of jaundice are:

Physiological (normal) jaundice: Most babies experience this mild jaundice at 2 to 4 days old because their liver is still maturing; it goes away in 1 or 2 weeks.

What should you do? This form usually corrects as baby's liver matures.

Breastfeeding jaundice: Baby isn't getting enough breast milk. It's not your breast milk that's the problem; but baby isn't getting enough fluid to pee and poop and get rid of the bilirubin.

What should you do? Pump and feed your baby all of the breast milk you're able to express. If needed, supplement with formula. Your doctor may also recommend phototherapy. This is when your baby is placed under lights for short periods of time. Light exposure helps degrade the bilirubin so it is excreted through poop.

Breast milk jaundice: In 1 to 2 percent of breastfed babies, jaundice is caused by an enzyme found in breast milk that makes the bilirubin level rise. It starts at 3 to 5 days old and improves over 3 to 12 weeks. It's not harmful to your baby.

What should you do? Your pediatrician may ask you to stop breastfeeding for a few days in order to assess; protect your milk supply by pumping or hand expressing every 3 to 4 hours. (You can feed this milk to your baby.) Even if it's confirmed that the jaundice is related to your milk, you should be able to return to breastfeeding as it's your milk increasing the bilirubin levels, not baby's inability to excrete it. As their liver matures, your baby will be able to get rid of the excess bilirubin on their own.

Blood group incompatibility (Rh or ABO problems): If you and your baby have different blood types, then your body might produce antibodies that destroy baby's red blood cells. This creates a sudden buildup of bilirubin in your baby's blood. This can be resolved by you receiving Rh immune-globulin injections during your pregnancy.

What should you do? Your pediatrician may take a small blood sample to measure the bilirubin level or monitor your baby to recommend treatment. A blood transfusion could be recommended to address severe jaundice that hasn't responded to other treatments.

BABY CARE

Now that we've taken a thorough look at nourishing your baby, let's move on to the other basic elements of baby care. I know it's a lot to take in. When everything is so new, every little thing can feel like a big deal. In this section, we'll take it step by step, from typical newborn appearance and clothing priorities to diapering and bathing. My hope is to set you up to make the transition to caring for your baby as simple as possible. You'll get the hang of it, and soon you and your baby will fall into a rhythm together—and caring for your baby will be completely natural.

Normal Newborn Appearance and Happenings

A lot of baby care is paying attention to what's going on with her; just simply observing her body and her movements and reactions can really help you know what to do. The trouble is, most of us have had very little experience with a newborn before we have one of our own! In that case, how can we know what normal appearance or behavior is? Luckily you have me, and I have this handy chart to help you learn about your new baby.

What Is It?	What Does It Look or Sound Like?	What's Going On?
Swelling	Puffy skin, especially around the face.	In the first few days of life, a newborn baby may appear swollen from her journey through the birth canal. The pressure and squeezing of that process can lead to swelling, leaving your newborn's eyelids temporarily puffy or swollen.
Vernix	A thick, white, waxy substance covering the skin.	The vernix protects the skin in utero and is deeply protective and moisturizing after birth as well. If your baby retains any vernix after birth, definitely delay his first bath so he can reap its benefits!
Head molding	Baby's head is misshapen, even a little cone-like.	Your baby's skull hasn't yet fused, so that she can make her way through the birth canal. This will smooth out as she grows, but the plates won't actually fully fuse for at least a year.
Stork bites	Small pink patches on the skin, usually found on the face or neck.	Found on only about one-third of newborns, stork bites (also called angel kisses) are temporary birthmarks, which fade by the time baby is six months old.

What Is It?	What Does It Look or Sound Like?	What's Going On?
Lanugo	Soft, peach-fuzz hair, sometimes covering the whole body, sometimes found in patches.	Lanugo, more common in premature babies, will wear off or fall off after the first weeks of life. Don't worry—baby won't look like a wolverine forever.
Swollen genitals	Baby's genital area and even breast tissue are swollen. Girls may have discharge, including blood.	Swollen tissue and discharge are all due to the surging hormone levels during birth. All of these conditions self-regulate and decrease in the days following birth.
Gagging	Baby may cough and gag.	Your baby is just clearing extra fluid and mucus from her lungs and throat. If it seems excessive, try using a bulb syringe—your hospital will give you one and show you how to use it.
Jerky movements	Arms and legs move in spasmodic, jerking motions.	It will take your baby a while to get the muscular control needed to make fluid motions. For now, her immature nervous system makes her movements pretty shaky.

>>>

What Is It?	What Does It Look or Sound Like?	What's Going On?
Meconium	Black, tar-like bowel movements.	Baby's first stools will be thick and black. Her stools will change to a mustard-like yellow within the first few days.
Weight loss	Baby appears thinner than at birth.	Babies lose up to 10 percent of their birth weight in the days following birth. They usually regain weight after seven to ten days, but speak to your pediatrician if you have weight concerns.
Periodic or loud breathing	A pause in the breath pattern.	New babies tend to breath super-fast, then take a deep breath. They breathe through the nose, allowing them to simultaneously breathe and feed.
Spit-up	Small amounts of regurgitated milk.	Babies typically spit up from swallowed air, so burping is essential. That said, some babies spit up more than others, and it's very common. The good news is, it doesn't seem to bother your baby—it just means more laundry for you.

What Is It?	What Does It Look or Sound Like?	What's Going On?
Cyanosis	Blue or gray coloring on the hands and feet.	Most common in the hours following birth, cyanosis has to do with circulation and oxygenation of the blood. New babies have poor circulation to their hands and feet; this will improve over a few weeks. If you're seeing a blue coloring many hours or days or months after birth, use socks or a hat. As long as your baby's lips and tongue are pink, no worries about the discolored extremities; it should disappear with warming.
Blotchy skin	Dry, peeling, or patchy-looking skin.	Your baby's skin is adjusting to her new environment. A gentle, baby-friendly oil, like grapeseed, can be helpful.
Nursing blister	White, blister-like skin on the lips.	It may look painful or irritated (it's actually not), but a nursing blister happens to be a sign of a good latch.
Cross-eyed	Baby may look cross-eyed or like he has a lazy eye.	Typically not an indication of vision problems, a cross-eyed appearance usually straightens out by three or four months of age.

>>>

What Is It?	What Does It Look or Sound Like?	What's Going On?
Moro reflex	Baby's arms suddenly go flying into the air and she looks extremely startled.	Your baby was born with many primitive reflexes; this is one of them. Swaddling can help keep her arms down, which will help keep her asleep.
Rooting	Baby opens her mouth and turns her head toward anything close by.	Another of her primitive reflexes at work; this one means baby is looking for something to eat!
Cradle cap	Scaly dry skin appears in patches or covers baby's scalp.	Cradle cap is completely harmless and doesn't bother your baby; still, you may want to try to remove it. Using baby oil and a soft brush is the best way to deal with cradle cap. Never pick at it or scratch it.
Swollen breasts	In both girls and boys the breasts might appear enlarged.	It's due to estrogen exposure in the uterus during your pregnancy. It can persist for several months after birth. Sometimes the breasts become engorged and drain a white liquid known as "witch's milk."
Vaginal discharge	Milky white liquid is discharged from the vagina.	Girls can have a milky vaginal discharge in the first few weeks of life that can even be blood-tinged. This is from exposure to high levels of estrogen during your pregnancy.

Miles and Miles

Your little baby sure does a sleep a lot—but that doesn't mean she's lazy. In fact, she's hard at work growing and developing. She's going to reach several developmental milestones before she's one month old! Here are some of the things your baby will get to in her first four weeks (get the camera!):

- Focuses on your face for short periods

- Holds head up for a few seconds when on tummy

- Sees objects 7 to 18 inches [17 to 46 cm] away

- Recognizes different smells (such as her mother's milk versus another's)

- Hears and recognizes familiar noises and voices

- Tastes all flavors (although prefers sweet)

Clothing

You may have already started venturing down the rabbit hole of babies' and children's clothing. There are so many great, cute-as-could-be options out there and in so many different price points. My advice, when it comes to your newborn, is to put all of that on hold and focus on a few different dressing priorities. You can go wild with adorableness once baby is a few more months old.

Material Your baby's skin is thinner and more sensitive than adult skin, so what you put next to it is important. Always go for natural fibers—cotton, merino, linen—and if it's within your budget, consider buying organic. Cotton crops are actually one of the largest consumers of pesticides worldwide—it's worth trying to avoid it. If cost is a concern, try limiting organic cottons to the base layer (closest to baby's skin). Always make sure to wash new clothing before dressing baby.

Temperature Babies have a tough time regulating their body temperature, so you'll want to think about the month and climate in which yours will be born. This goes both ways: Babies can become cold very easily, but they can also become overheated. In general, a good rule of thumb is that your baby should wear what you wear, plus one layer. The best way to help baby regulate his temperature is to get plenty of time skin to skin.

Umbilical cord Your baby's umbilical cord stump can actually persist for quite a while, so you'll want loose clothing that doesn't stick or snag this area. I love kimono tops for this reason. A kimono top and some footed pants are a perfect newborn uniform. Make sure to keep pants fairly low-slung at this point—the elastic band shouldn't interfere with the umbilical cord either. (See Cord Care in the Diapering section, page 378.)

Mittens and booties If their baby will tolerate them, some mothers choose to use mittens in the first few weeks or months. A baby's herky-jerky arm motions and propensity to bring hands to face can lead to little cuts and scrapes on his face. In my experience, booties and socks almost never stay put—I always recommend footed pants or footed onesies instead.

For a full list of what you'll need—and some recommended brands—check The Goods, on page 406.

Diapering

Newborn babies need a diaper change very frequently—think ten or more times per day—so the great news is, even if you aren't very experienced with diapers, you'll get up to speed. Quickly. This may not be the most eagerly anticipated part of new motherhood, but you may even establish a nice changing table routine with your baby. You never know where you'll find a new opportunity to connect.

However, in the early days and weeks, the changing table space can really get babies worked up and activated, crying and squirming. Try implementing some type of ritual to soothe your baby. Maybe you'll sing a certain song, tell her stories, or describe the day. Whatever it is, keep it consistent, and your baby will soon start to associate this time with a closeness to you.

Diaper 101 All diapers consist of two essential ingredients: a soft, absorbent inner layer for liquids and a waterproof outer "shell" to keep in solids. There are many different styles and variations on this theme—getting to know which is right for your baby will depend on fit and a bit of trial and error. Think of diaper fit like a pair of jeans: Some just seem to be tailor-made for your specific rear end. For this reason, I wouldn't stock up on a ton of the cutest patterned diapers you can find—try to get packs from a handful of different companies and see what seems to work best on your baby.

Cloth or disposable? Ultimately, this is going to be a personal question and depends entirely on your priorities. Cloth diapers create less waste, are gentle on baby's skin, and can save your family money over time. That said, you'll be adding a lot of (yes, pretty smelly) laundry to the load, and they can be more expensive up front. There are cloth diaper laundering services that can help make things a little easier. Disposables are convenient, and there are biodegradable and sensitive-skin options out there. They are also less expensive than a diaper service, depending on the brand you buy. A third option is a hybrid diaper system, which incorporates a disposable liner into a reusable cloth diaper cover.

Movements Your baby's first bowel movements, called meconium, will be sticky and tarry black. By day 2 or 3 her poops will begin to look brown or brown-green in color, with the consistency of mustard, eventually turning a more yellow color by day 4 or 5. Breastfed babies may poop after every feed, and the poop may even have curds. Formula-fed babies may produce only one to three stools per day, and they may be darker.

Wipes Standard moist cleansing wipes shouldn't be used on a newborn baby for at least the first two weeks. Their skin is simply too sensitive, even if the wipe is mostly water or marked for sensitive skin. Instead, use water on a cotton swab with a bit of grapeseed oil to remove anything particularly difficult like meconium. You can keep grapeseed oil in a pump bottle on your changing table. You can also make your own homemade wipes with the recipe that follows. When you do choose wipes, try to choose ones that are organic or have very few moisturizing ingredients.

Elimination communication EC is a diaper-free method for dealing with baby's waste; it is a common practice worldwide where the ability to clean or dispose of diapers is very limited. This method requires paying close attention to your baby's cues to urinate or have a bowel movement. Parents look out for and observe certain cues from their baby to know that they need to urinate or make a bowel movement; then they hold their baby over a sink or potty. *The Diaper-Free Baby: The Natural Toilet Training Alternative* by Christine Gross-Loh is a good place to start to learn more.

Circumcision care Your baby's circumcision should heal in seven to ten days. Circumcision is considered a very safe procedure and risk of infection is very low. With each diaper change, clean around the penis area, apply petroleum jelly (so the wound doesn't stick to his diaper), and cover with a small piece of medical gauze. It should heal on its own, naturally. A clear yellow crust, raw appearance, and small amount of bleeding are normal. Call your doctor if your son doesn't make a wet diaper within six to eight hours after the procedure; if the wound bleeds excessively; if redness, swelling, or discharge doesn't resolve after a week; or if he has a temperature of 100.4°F [38°C] or higher.

Cord care In addition to avoiding snug clothing, there are a handful of other ways to help your baby's umbilical cord heal properly and eventually fall off anywhere from five to twenty-one days after birth. Clean around the stump, but never get it directly wet; fold down the top front of your baby's diaper to prevent irritation; and avoid creams and powders around the stump. Call your pediatrician if the stump is actively bleeding, the base is swollen or red, the cord is oozing a foul-smelling white or yellow discharge, or your baby has a fever.

··

Simple Homemade Wipes

½ cup [120 ml] water
1 tablespoon organic aloe vera
1 tablespoon witch hazel
2 tablespoons grapeseed oil

40 large cotton pads (typically
   used for removing makeup)
Wipes warmer

Combine the water, aloe vera, witch hazel, and oil in a bowl. Add the pads to the solution to saturate. Then gently press to remove the excess water and place in the wipes warmer. You'll probably need to make a batch of these once a week. If you'd like to make these reusable, swap out the cotton pads for muslin baby towels.

··

Bathing

Bath time may conjure childhood memories of rubber duckies, toy boats, and fun splashing, but bathing a newborn or young baby is a much more mellow experience. In fact, your baby will want you to keep things as slow and relaxed as possible so she can become familiar with the experience. Much like establishing a ritual for the changing table, this can be as simple as a song you always sing at the bath or a retelling of the day's events. Don't get too overly complicated with it: It's important that the ritual is also something you will like doing day in and out. Let's look at the two ways you'll bathe your baby in these early days.

Sponge bath While your baby's umbilical cord stump is still attached, you will be sponge bathing her exclusively. The truth is, besides a little spit-up, there's not much to clean (your diapering routine handles all of that). These early-days sponge baths are as much about familiarity and practice as they are about getting your baby squeaky clean. Here are a few things to keep in mind for sponge bathing:

- You will need a hooded towel, bowl of warm water, soft washcloths, mild baby soap (no soap before two weeks—just water, because their skin is sensitive), and a fresh diaper and clothes.

- Wrap your baby in her towel; uncover only the part of her body that you intend to clean, tucking it back into the towel when you're finished.

- Dip your washcloth in the water and start with her face: Gently wipe over her eyes, around her mouth, and especially under her chin and neck, where spit-up and milk can accumulate.

- Put a pea-size amount of soap on a washcloth and clean your baby's body, taking extra care in folds and creases, like between fingers and toes and around the genital area. If needed, use another small pea of soap to wash baby's hair and scalp, then rinse with a small amount of water.

- Dry off your baby and use a soft-bristled baby brush on her hair. Then just diaper and clothe her.

Tub Once your baby's umbilical cord stump has fully fallen off, she'll be ready to move into her tub. Look for a baby tub with head and neck support that can help prevent slipping (wet babies are very slippery). The general process for bathing your baby will be the same as for the sponge bath, with these additional tips:

- Fill the tub with only a few inches of water, at most 3 inches [7.5 cm]. The water should be warm, but not hot. Test the temperature with your elbow or a thermometer (many baby thermometers can also measure water temperature).

- Wash baby's face first without any soap; shampoo your baby's scalp last, so she can stay warm longer.

- Place your baby's towel on the ground or a nearby flat surface. Gently lift baby from the tub and rest her on her towel, then wrap her up and dry her off. This technique is easier than trying to dry your tiny baby in mid-air.

- Never keep the water running when your baby is in the tub, and never leave baby unattended in the bath.

Baby Massage

For soothing and bonding with your baby, it doesn't get much better than baby massage. A widespread practice in India as part of Ayurvedic medicine, baby massage has also been popular historically in China, New Zealand, Africa, and the Caribbean as well. These days, it's gaining popularity in the Western world as the importance and soothing power of touch is starting to become better known. Baby massage has many benefits, including the regulation of the circulatory, nervous, and immune systems. It also tends to deeply soothe babies, which ultimately helps them sleep better. What follows is a step-by-step guide to baby massage, but feel free to experiment with what seems to work with your baby. These guidelines can really be a jumping-off point.

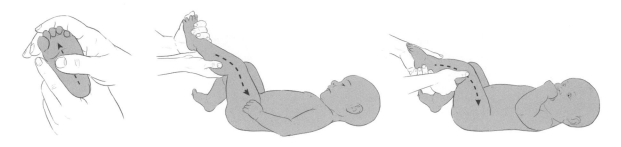

Demonstration of massage steps 2 and 3

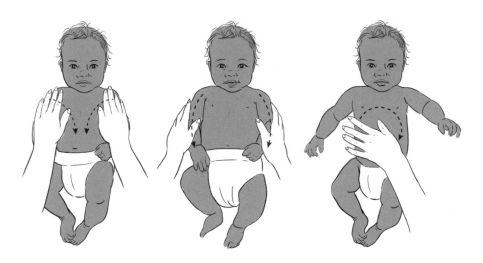

Demonstration of massage steps 4 and 5

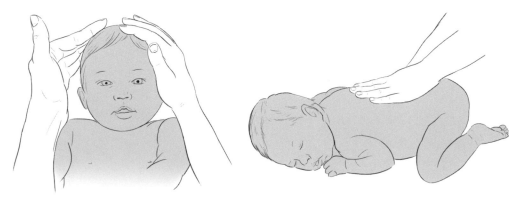

Demonstration of massage steps 6 and 7

Step 1

Adjust your environment as you would want for your own massage. The room should be warm, and your baby should be quiet, well rested, and alert.

Step 2

Begin by gently massaging your baby's feet from heel to toes.

Step 3

Continue by massaging each of his legs in an upward movement. Flex your baby's knee against his belly to help expel any gas.

Step 4

Moving on to the upper body, gently massage from your baby's shoulders inward toward his chest. Then, stroke down his arms. Avoid his hands— you don't want him to end up ingesting the oil.

Step 5

If your baby has a fully belly, avoid massaging there. Otherwise, make very gentle circular motions over his belly area.

Step 6

You can use your fingertips to very gently massage your baby's face, stroking from the center of his forehead around his eyes and across his cheeks.

Step 7

Finally, if your baby is comfortable on his tummy, you can flip him over and do long strokes along his back, from the nape of his neck and down each leg.

A few notes: Choose a massage oil that is gentle, organic, and fragrance-free. Grapeseed or coconut oil are perfect. Additionally, always be respectful of your baby's touch preferences. You may have high hopes for massage with your baby, but it's important to put his cues first. If he cries, fusses, or resists, end the session and try again another time.

SOOTHING

Besides breastfeeding, handling a crying baby is most new mothers' most anxious anticipation. In the past, if you happened to find yourself holding a baby in the throes of unhappiness, all you'd have to do is hand her back to her mother. And now that mother is you. I get it, but here's the truth: Your baby has very few ways to communicate her needs to you. Besides those oh-so-subtle cues, crying is her best way of getting your attention. And here's another thing I know to be true: You will, eventually, come to find your own unique way to soothe your baby; all mothers do.

The Five S's

In 2002, Dr. Harvey Karp released his book *The Happiest Baby on the Block*, which announced his theory of the fourth trimester—and his techniques on how to cope with it. These days, the theory of the fourth trimester and Dr. Karp's Five S's are so well known that your pediatrician may even hand you a leaflet about how to do it. It works.

The basic premise is that, because of humans' complicated and large brains, babies are born "too early" in order to fit through the pelvis. He argues that the period of time from birth to three or four months—the so-called "fourth trimester"—is the final period of a baby's gestation. For this reason, the soothing techniques that work best at this time aren't the same as at other times in a baby's life. In fact, Dr. Karp's soothing techniques, the Five S's, are all meant to mimic life in the womb.

Each of the Five S's can soothe your baby individually, but in certain cases, or if your baby is particularly upset, you may want to do all five, building up from one to the next (and in the order presented here).

Swaddling A (surprisingly) tight swaddle helps your baby feel secure, like she did in the womb.

Side holding Hold your baby on her side to prevent her startle reflex, which kicks in when she's on her back.

Shushing Babies love loud white noise (think vacuum cleaners, air conditioners, or blenders) because they mimic the sounds they're used to in the womb. You can "shhhh" into your baby's ear or try a sound machine. You'll just have to make sure it gets loud enough.

Swinging Life in the womb is full of movement, so resting statically can be a little jarring for your baby. Slower rocking is fine most of the time, but if she's at level 10, a stronger and more rhythmic jostle is best. It can be tough to get the hang of this (after all, you should never violently shake your baby); to see what this should be like, check YouTube for videos of Dr. Karp soothing babies.

Sucking Your baby has a strong need to suck, and it can be deeply calming for her. Offering her a pacifier or the tip of your finger can be just the thing to finally calm her down.

The Soothing Circuit

Now that you know about diapers, gas, feeding, and the Five S's, you're ready for the Soothing Circuit. Essentially, you're checking off a list of possibilities for the causes of fussiness: Is it a diaper? Nope. Is it gas? Nope. Eventually you'll build up to the Five S's, where you're soothing a baby whose needs are met but who just needs a little more TLC. Call it #fourthtrimesterproblems.

There is one topic in the Soothing Circuit that may not have occurred to you, and that is to scan your baby. Little things like itchy clothing tags, a stray hair or loose thread wrapped around a toe, or anything that could be pulling or tugging on your baby can seriously distress him. Therefore, the last step before implementing the Five S's is to scan your baby for any outlying irritators.

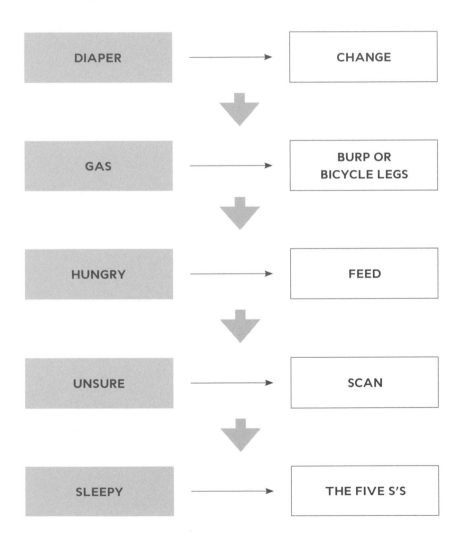

A Few Words on Pacifiers

While wonderfully soothing for your baby, pacifiers shouldn't be used until after two to three weeks of life. During that time, your milk supply is still being established, and if your baby's hunger is curbed by pacifier use, your supply may drop below what's needed. For this reason, sucking is the last soothing method of the Five S's—used well after you've already checked to see if your baby is hungry. A few more tips about pacifiers:

- Look for cylindrical-shaped pacifiers, which are best for breastfed babies.

- Don't use pacifiers in the half-hour to hour before your next feed, so that you can observe hunger cues.

- Don't use a pacifier during a growth spurt, which is a time when it's important for you to establish your milk supply.

- Don't offer a pacifier if your baby is already relaxed and happy.

- If your baby is sleeping well and easily soothed without one, no need to even bother with a pacifier.

SLEEP

Newborn babies sleep in half-hour to four-hour stretches, waking to feed. What's more, they'll often take their most continuous sleep right in the middle of the day. This can certainly leave you disoriented (take a look back at Chapter Eleven for methods for dealing with fatigue), but it is more or less how things will be for at least a few months. Most babies are not ready to transition to a more adult sleep pattern (say, five or more continuous nighttime sleep hours) until they're at least three months old. At about twelve weeks, your baby's brain will begin to secrete the hormone melatonin, which will help her consolidate her sleep periods and settle at night. Until then, your baby will exhibit three distinct sleep states: deep sleep, light sleep, and drowsiness. In deep sleep, your baby is getting her most restorative, growth sleep. She is still and calm; her breathing is rhythmic. She doesn't need anything at this time and shouldn't be wakened. In light sleep, your baby's eyes are closed, but active under her eyelids. She may turn her head to root, move her arms and legs, and respond to noise. If you feed her in this state, she may fall back into a deep sleep. Though drowsiness is technically a waking state, it's still related to your baby's sleep state. She could exhibit sleep cues, like yawning and rubbing her eyes. Her breathing may be irregular, and she may react to stimuli very slowly. If you hope she'll sleep, try soothing her by rocking, shushing, or singing quietly and feeding her. If you want to rouse her, try something active like talking to her, walking around, or dancing. Generally speaking, your baby's pattern of sleeping and waking in short bits are what she needs in order to gain weight and grow. While your baby is hard at work eating, sleeping, digesting, and getting hungry again, there are several ways you can work with your baby to ease through this transition.

Cosleeping For the first several months of your baby's life, it can be helpful to have her "room in" or cosleep, which means she'll sleep in your room in a small crib or bassinet. There are also beds called "cosleepers" available, which are essentially three-sided bassinets that attach to the side of your bed. Studies show that breastfeeding mothers tend to get more sleep while cosleeping, as feeding becomes much easier and less disruptive to your own sleep. Cosleeping also can reduce the risk of sudden infant death syndrome (SIDS) because you are more likely to subconsciously sense if your baby's health is in danger and wake up because of the close proximity.

Bed-sharing A step beyond cosleeping, bed-sharing means just that: Your baby will sleep in your bed with you. There are certain safety risks associated with bed-sharing (namely, sleepy parents rolling onto their baby), but the practice can be safe given a few very important measures.

For more information on both cosleeping and bed-sharing, read Professor James J. McKenna's (of Notre Dame's Mother-Baby Behavioral Sleep Laboratory) book *Sleeping with Your Baby: A Parent's Guide to Cosleeping* or visit his personal website.

Safety Checklist for Baby's Sleep Environment

All sleep:

- Always put baby to sleep on her back.

- Sleep surface should be firm.

- Bedding and swaddling blankets should all be taut—no loose fabric.

- The bed environment shouldn't have any pillows, toys, or blankets, even if they are soft.

- Babies should never sleep on a sofa, chair, or other surface where she could become wedged.

Bed-sharing:

- Smokers should not bed-share with their babies.

- Premature babies or babies with a low birth weight should not bed-share.

- Do not bed-share with your baby if you have had alcohol, sedatives, or any drugs.

- Baby should bed-share with parents only—no older siblings.

- Do not swaddle your baby while bed-sharing.

- Any long hair should be tied up.

The right light Until birth, your baby lived in total darkness—no wonder he has no clue about day and night! You can help him understand the difference with a few subtle changes to the environment. For instance, make sure he sees a lot of bright natural sunlight during day hours and little to no artificial light at night. That doesn't mean you necessarily have to keep your house pitch black in the evening; very dim lighting or candles will do the trick.

Your routine The best way to acclimate your baby to the rhythm of life outside the womb is to take her along in your daily routine. Whether that means bringing her along to the grocery store or wearing her in a sling or carrier wrap while you do the dishes, social cues can actually be a low-stress way to get her into the flow.

Common Challenges, Concerns, and Warning Signs

A newborn in the house is cause for joy—but can come with an equal weight of anxiety as well. Here are a few common challenges, areas of concern, and warning signs that may (or may not) come up.

Abnormal temperature If your baby is under six months old and has an abnormal temperature, call his pediatrician immediately. An abnormal temperature is anything above 99.5°F [37.5°C] or under 97.4°F [36.3°C]. Both can be signs of an infection; the lower temperature can be a sign of a bacterial infection.

Yellow coloring If your baby's face, chest, or whites of his eyes have a yellow tint, this is a sign of jaundice. While your baby was in utero, your liver helped regulate levels of bilirubin in his blood. After birth, levels can surge and give a yellowish tint to the skin. Nursing frequently typically does the trick, but speak to your pediatrician about care procedures, or if the coloring persists or gets worse. See Hello, Yellow (page 368).

Problems feeding A baby who is not feeding at least seven or eight times in a twenty-four-hour period is not feeding well. Especially at risk are babies struggling with weight gain, babies who were premature, and babies with jaundice. This is a reason to call your pediatrician.

Fewer diapers If your baby isn't making as many soiled diapers as she should be, she isn't getting enough food, and you should contact your pediatrician and/or lactation consultant immediately. In her first week, she should make as many wet diapers as days since birth (three diapers at three days of age) and six or more wet diapers per twenty-four-hour period after the first week. Your baby should not go more than twenty-four hours without a bowel movement (until about six months old).

Difficulty breathing If your baby has blue lips, flared nostrils, or deep indentations in his chest, or appears to be struggling to breathe, call 9-1-1 immediately, then your doctor.

A SIDS Primer

SIDS, or sudden infant death syndrome, is admittedly a scary prospect. Know that the chances of your baby dying of SIDS are actually very low, and there are some very concrete things you can do to protect your baby from SIDS and lower the risk of its happening to your family.

What Is SIDS?

SIDS is the sudden death of a baby, seemingly by suffocation, but with inconclusive autopsy results. One theory is that babies with SIDS have lower levels of serotonin, which controls breathing and heart rate during sleep and so makes it more difficult for the baby to wake if something is going wrong. Whatever the cause, new guidelines for sleep safety have dramatically reduced the already-small chances of SIDS.

Tips to Prevent SIDS

Although there is no "cure" for SIDS, and there is nothing parents can do to entirely prevent it, statistics show that implementing the following safety protocol has helped diminish the number of cases of SIDS.

- Always put your baby to sleep on her back.

- Use a firm mattress and tightly fitting sheets (never any loose fabric).

- There shouldn't be anything else in the crib besides your baby. No bumper, no pillow, no lovey; nothing else.

- Prevent your baby from overheating. Don't overdress her, and keep her room at 68° to 72°F [20° to 22°C].

- Keep baby's room well ventilated. Use a fan if it feels stuffy.

- When your baby is at least two or three weeks old, if she is well fed but still fretful, offer her a pacifier. (But don't stress if she doesn't take it.)

- Cosleep with your baby for the first three to six months.

BONDING THROUGH PLAY

She's fed, she's slept, and maybe you've had the chance to do the same. Now, what can you do with those few extra minutes before that flow starts up again? Play. Keep in mind there is no right or wrong way to do this. In fact, every time you hold, diaper, or just simply look at your baby you are engaging, playing, and bonding. You might have felt an immediate bond with your baby the instant you held her in your arms or you might discover you're struggling to find a recognizable connection a few weeks in. Wherever you are in this spectrum is OK. Be gentle on yourself and surrender to your own mothering pace. Bonding with your baby takes time and you have your whole life to nurture that bond. That said, the activities below will help foster that bond and help you discover a playful way to interact with your baby and positively impact their brain development in the first three months. You can find recommendations on where to find these items in the Resources section (see page 415).

Gaze with intention. Start with gazing at your baby directly in her eyes. It's a simple and engaging form of play. Research has shown that newborn babies prefer to look at faces over any other kind of interaction or toy. In fact, they prefer to look at faces that are smiling and intentionally responsive to their actions. Also, within the first week your baby already recognizes you from strangers and prefers you. All you need is a few minutes. You can lie your baby on her back, hold her in your arms, or you can even do it while you breastfeed or feed her.

Tummy time. Once your baby's umbilical cord falls off you can start by gently rolling baby into the tummy-down position after being placed on her back. Tummy time helps strengthen her head, neck, and upper body muscles and prevents flat head syndrome. You can do it on the floor or a firm surface using a blanket; make sure to lie down next to or watch your baby while you do this. Alternatively, you can simply place her on your chest while you're in a semi-reclined position, which is less horizontal (and less scary) for baby and is a nice bonus snuggle for you. You'll probably find that the best time to do this will usually be right after diaper changes. Only do it for 2 to 5 minutes at a time or as long as your baby feels comfortable. Shift your baby over onto her back if she starts to appear tired, rests her face on the blanket or your chest, or starts to cry. If you end tummy time before she cries or becomes fatigued, the sooner she begins to acclimate and enjoy being on her tummy.

BABY-WEARING

Imagine going through your day, running errands, meeting friends, going for a walk, or even just moving around the house with your little baby sleeping tucked against your chest. Baby-wearing is a sweet way to navigate these early weeks, and there are also some strong pragmatic reasons for wearing your baby in a carrier or wrap. Baby-wearing is growing in popularity as new mothers come to realize the convenience and intense bonding that comes with the practice. In addition, there's also lots of scientific evidence to support the benefits of wearing your baby.

Less crying. This one is simple: Babies love being close to their mothers and cry far less when they are worn. Don't fret if it seems like your baby doesn't like to be in her carrier. Because it's new—and she can sense you're probably a little anxious about it—your baby may fuss a bit when you first try her in her sling, wrap, or carrier. My advice? Strap or wrap her in, make sure she appears comfortable, and then go for a walk around the block. Most times, your baby will be content and/or asleep by the time you complete the loop.

More learning. Babies who spend most of their time being worn are often in a state of quiet alertness rather than fussing and crying. That means that they have a better opportunity to take in their world and interact with their mother—and are therefore often far more advanced than their non-worn buddies.

Carry On

There are many different types of carriers out there, but to my mind, these are all you need.

A soft wrap. This is essentially a long piece of fabric that you wrap around you and your baby. Especially when your baby is small and you don't need much in the way of ergonomics and back support, these are a great option, as they can really feel like a second skin.

Structured carrier. Somewhat like a backpack, these are great because of their durability. Some models are very versatile: You can wear baby tummy-to-tummy, tummy-to-back, on your side, and on your back. Look for carriers that are easy to put on (not too many straps and buckles) and that promote the "happy hips" position for baby, which positions knees above hips and is best for their comfort.

For both carrier styles, use this checklist to ensure proper wearing safety:

- **Snug:** Your baby should be snug to your chest.

- **Visible:** You should be able to see your baby at all times.

- **Kissable:** You should be able to kiss the top of your baby's head. If not, he's too low.

- **Chin off chest:** To keep his airways free and clear, your baby's chin should not slump onto his chest.

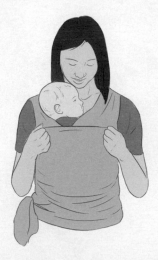 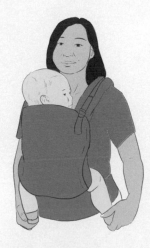

Soft wrap carrier   Soft structured carrier

Safe to explore. Consider this: A newborn baby lying on his back in a crib hears a loud noise and is startled. His Moro reflex goes off, his arms fly into the air, and he starts to cry. In comparison, a baby being worn with his mother hears a loud noise, but because he feels safe tucked against you (and is upright, preventing the Moro reflex), he looks to see where the noise came from. From the comforting safety of your chest, he can look around and explore his world (even if it's a little loud).

Less gas. After you feed your baby, it's best to keep her upright for ten minutes so that she can easily burp or pass gas (which is tougher to do if she's lying down). This is a great time to hold her in your carrier or wrap—and to fix yourself a snack as well.

Easier regulation. A baby who spends his time held against her mother's chest learns a lot from her. He listens to her heart beating, her breathing, and other bodily noises and feels her warmth. This helps him become familiar with these functions in himself. Additionally, most wraps and carriers can be used as a breastfeeding support, so your baby will be able to more easily sate himself and fall into a rhythm of being carried and being fed.

Socialization. This may seem counterintuitive, but a baby who spends her days strapped onto Mama is actually learning early social skills as she sees and hears everything that her mother does in a day. From this intimate vantage point, your baby can hear the rhythm of your voice, feel the way you move, and see how you and your partner interact with other people and your environment.

Mama Mantra
Slow down
and create space for
quiet moments.

Epilogue:

Finding Your New Normal

———

Way back in the beginning of this book, I observed how your first pregnancy and, especially, the birth are, in many ways, the first time you'll act as a mother. Over the past ten months, you have made so many new and import-ant decisions about your health, your self-care, your baby, your emotional landscape—looking inward, while staying curious about new information and surroundings. And now here you are, an actual mother of a brand-new baby! After nine or so months, you may feel like it's already been a long journey, but really, it's only just begun.

I understand that may be daunting for you to hear. You may worry whether you're up to the task of raising a whole human being to adulthood. Just about any big, long-term responsibility can feel overwhelming if you zoom out too far. You may have a little inner voice feeding you critical, unhelpful self-doubt, or actual people in your life who make you feel like you don't know what you're doing. I encourage you to stay curious and let each moment, each day, each year unfold on its own. When your baby is ten, you too will have grown up ten years; when she's eighteen, you will have known and supported her for eighteen years. Your lives will grow together in tandem, not all at once. Just as you've been practicing since the beginning of your pregnancy, you will continue to find your most powerful strength in your own intuition.

The truth is, now, as ever: You've got this.

Throughout this book, I've encouraged you to look within yourself for the answers to your toughest questions. Using your internal compass, your personal intuition, you'll be able to navigate the first step of this journey. As you venture further into motherhood, continue to revisit these self-assuring thoughts. Use this book as a resource and an affirmation if you need to—or continue to forge ahead on your own.

To close, I'd like to offer you some affirmations to keep in mind as you move into your new normal—motherhood.

Be gentle on yourself and others. It's so easy to fall into a cycle of judgment, thinking you should be more like another mother, or your family like some other family. Be as patient with others as you would have them be for you. (Judge not, lest ye be judged.) Be understanding; we each do things our own way. If you wonder if a friend will take your advice (about your go-to product or a book you think everyone should read—maybe even this one!), try to release yourself from their decision, their judgment, their right to choose otherwise. Instead, feel compassion and assume that we are all doing the best we can do with the information we have.

Make time for yourself. Be assertive about your need for self-care, which can quickly diminish when you begin caring for another. Taking good care of yourself will enable you to take the best care of your baby.

Make time for your partner. It's so important to nurture the love and connection that brought your baby into your lives.

Go slow and soak it all in. Many times, mothers understand how special and fleeting it all is only once their baby is older. Take in every moment, starting now. These times simply won't come again; enjoy them.

Allow and welcome support. Surround yourself with supportive individuals—those people who help out literally and those who just lift you up in indescribable ways. You'll want more and more friends, family members, and colleagues who come to you without judgment, who just want to be there for you. Allow them to help you; seek them out any time you need the reinforcement. You're not expected to have all the answers to everything. Be open and welcome help. (That said, it's OK to know when to nod your head at unwelcome advice and let it fade away.)

Stay playful. Being a mother is a time to remember what you loved about being a child. Silly songs, art projects, getting outdoors, even things like making funny faces—indulge in the simple joy of childhood.

Speak your truth. I've noticed that mothers don't like to speak up when things are going well—they may feel like they're bragging or that they'll jinx whatever great thing is happening (say, sleeping through the night) and it will stop. On the other hand, some women don't want to share what's been tough or admit it when things are difficult. This dialogue is open to all experiences and voices, as it should be. Letting your community in, no matter what your experience is, should and will be fruitful.

Establish your flow . . . Eventually, you'll find yourself in a solid rhythm with your baby. You'll feel that things are really working, that you have a handle on it. Live these moments to their fullest—use nap times and nighttimes as moments for self-care and projects: Journal, meditate, and recharge however you like to. These quiet moments can be points of inspiration.

. . . then let it go. The first year is very much a year of quarters. As soon as you think you've got it, that you understand what's going on with your baby, he's going to go through a developmental surge and is going to change. You're going to feel like you're starting right back at the beginning again. That is normal and something to anticipate. Go back to our conversation about birth and revisit that sense of "choosing, then letting go"; try to remember what it felt like, waxing and waning with your contractions. Harness that energy of flexibility, and know that you will find your flow again. Flexibility, patience, and understanding are essential parts of the journey of motherhood.

Stay in touch with what works. In this book we've worked to help you support yourself through self-care and self-reflection throughout your pregnancy. Too often, after their baby arrives new mothers forget about all these wonderfully enriching rituals. Find ways to incorporate what we talk about in this book into your daily life with your baby. If your baby's crying triggers an irritated emotion, bring it back to POP and the Feelings Circle; revisit the Five-Minute Reboot while you're quietly breastfeeding your baby. Adjusting to the new moments and the scarcity of time will be tough, but if you are able, the self-affirmation will be deeply beneficial.

You did it, you're doing it, and you will continue to do it! Days with your baby will be full—of small victories and disappointments, joy and banality. What I really want for you to take away from this book is that mothering and motherhood can look so many different ways. The world needs more people tapping into their deepest intuition and mothering from a place that feels uniquely right for them. The more we do that—moving away from comparison, embracing our individuality—the better all of our experiences will be.

I'm thrilled for you, and I'm so proud of you.

Resources

THE GOODS

Over the years, my clients have been the best teachers. Working from their collective recommendations and my own scrupulous research, I've developed The Goods, a comprehensive shopping guide for soon-to-be and new mothers. Surprisingly, collecting everything that you need can be a cause of anxiety during this time—my hope is that this list will help ease some of that anxiety. There is a range of brands, from small businesses and boutique brands to big box stores, and a range of price points.

Pregnancy Goods

You don't need much during pregnancy, but here are a few essentials that will keep you comfortable during those months and well into the postpartum shift.

Wellness

Item	Brands	Tips
Prenatal vitamin	MegaFood: Baby and Me, Metagenics, Wellness Essentials Pregnancy	A food-based daily multivitamin that meets the daily recommended intake for both folate and vitamin D. I always recommend food-based supplements rather than synthetic.
Folate + vitamin D	Brand is less important; make sure to buy methl-folate (5-mthf), the bioavailable form (more on page 76)	Recently in *Drug and Therapeutics Bulletin*, a UK periodical, researchers have advised that daily prenatal multivitamins may not be necessary. The only components that are necessary are folate and vitamin D. Taken in conjunction with a well-rounded, nutritious diet (like the

Item	Brands	Tips
		recipes in this book!), you should have no trouble getting the nutrition you need for both you and your baby. This is a great conversation for you and your care provider.
Ginger	New Chapter	Up to 1 gram (1000 mg) daily; take in divided doses as needed for relief.
B6	Source Naturals	Also known for helping to relieve nausea and vomiting in pregnancy; consider taking 25 mg twice a day, morning and evening, to help manage your symptoms.
Probiotic	NatureWise Womens Love	Take one daily with food; store in the fridge.
Digestive enzymes	Rainbow Light Advanced Enzyme Optima	Especially potent in papaya enzyme supplements, these help healthy digestion and reduce inflammation.
Flower remedies	Bach's Original Flower Remedies: White Chestnut, Red Chestnut, Rescue Remedy Floracopeia	Flower infusions are safe and gentle forms of relief from many complaints, most notably anxiety and stress.
Magnesium (citrate or malate)	Natural Calm, Source Materials	An easy-to-use, natural powder formulation or capsule.
Epsom or magnesium salts	Epsoak	Great for a bath at the end of a long day or for soaking feet.

Item	Brands	Tips
Nettle leaf	Mountain Rose Herbs	Tends to be a popular item and can sell out; if you love the infusion, buy it in bulk.
Red raspberry leaf	Mountain Rose Herbs	Tends to be a popular item and can sell out; if you love the infusion, buy it in bulk.
Chamomile flower	Mountain Rose Herbs	Helps promote sleep and relaxation.
Hibiscus flower	Mountain Rose Herbs	Helps encourage fluid balance, alleviate occasional constipation, and promote proper circulation. It is commonly used in combination with lemon balm and St. John's wort for restlessness and occasional difficulty falling asleep.
Lemon balm leaf	Mountain Rose Herbs	Helps provide a sense of balance for the nervous system while it supports the immune system; it can also provide comfort for occasional digestive distress.
Lemon essential oil	Snow Lotus, Mountain Rose Herbs, Floracopeia	Helps reduce nausea; can also help manage stress.
Peppermint essential oil	Snow Lotus Aromatherapy, Mountain Rose Herbs, Floracopeia	Helps uplift and stimulate; eases sugar cravings and nausea.

Item	Brands	Tips
Lavender essential oil	Snow Lotus, Mountain Rose Herbs, Floracopeia	Helps reduce anxiety and anger and manage stress; promotes sleep.
Frankincense essential oil	Snow Lotus, Mountain Rose Herbs, Floracopeia	Helps ease anxiety and depression.
Mandarin/orange essential oil	Snow Lotus, Mountain Rose Herbs, Floracopeia	Helps relieve anxiety; promotes deep breathing.
Spikenard essential oil	Snow Lotus, Mountain Rose Herbs, Floracopeia	Helps relieve anxiety and fear; is calming and grounding.
Clary sage essential oil	Snow Lotus, Mountain Rose Herbs, Floracopeia	Helps relieves anger and stress.
Rose geranium essential oil	Snow Lotus, Mountain Rose Herbs, Floracopeia	Helps balance moods; relieves restlessness.
Sandalwood essential oil	Snow Lotus, Mountain Rose Herbs, Floracopeia	Eases stress, promotes deep breathing, can feel tranquilizing.
Neroli essential oil	Snow Lotus, Mountain Rose Herbs, Floracopeia	Helps lift mood; eases depression and distress.
Sweet almond oil or sesame seed oil	Life-flo (Organic), Mountain Rose Herbs, Floracopeia	This a carrier oil to blend your other oils with; if you are sensitive to nuts, avoid both and use grapeseed oil instead.

Apparel

Item	Brands	Tips
Maternity belt or band	Belly Bandit Upsie Belly, Preggers	Can be very helpful from Month Six onward.
Compression socks	Gabrialla, Preggers	Great for long car trips or flying, or on days when you're feeling more swollen.
Maternity clothes	Storq, Hatch, Blanqi, Zara, H&M, Target, or go vintage on sites like Etsy or look for clothing that has the ability to stretch and accommodate your body as it grows and changes.	Look for clothes that you'll wear through pregnancy and postpartum—that means tops that open for breastfeeding and anything you'd wear to feel comfortable and confident, even if your body is different than expected. I love loose dresses with buttons down the front allowing for easy access, or a kaftan.

Baby Goods

Apparel

Item (How Many)	Brands	Tips
Kimono tops (4) or side-snap tees	Giggle, Target, Carter's, Under the Nile, Polarn O. Pyret	Creates less friction on the umbilical cord stump, until it falls off. Combine tops with footed pants.
Tops and shirts (6)	Primary, H&M (organic), Giggle, Target	Stick with things that snap and don't need to be pulled over baby's head—makes for easier changing sessions.

Item (How Many)	Brands	Tips
Footed pants (4)	H&M, Giggle, Target, Carter's	Socks tend to never stay on for too long, so footed pants are a great alternative to keep those little feet warm.
Pants (4)	Primary, H&M, Giggle, Target	For warmer weather, after the first few weeks, footed pants aren't necessary
Onesies and jumpsuits (6)	Primary, H&M, Giggle, Target	Get both long-sleeved and short-sleeved onesies. Look for snap closures—makes for easy diaper changes.
Convertible gowns (3)	Giggle, Target, Under the Nile	Gathered at the hem, these gowns convert from pants to a cocoon for seamless play-to-nap transitions and diaper changes.
Sweaters and/ or jackets (2)	Primary, Patagonia	Depending on the time of year or climate, you might need two or more of these.
Socks and booties (3 pairs)	Primary, H&M, Giggle, Target	It's great to have a few, but you'll probably find that footed pants are your default.
Hats (4)	Carter's, Giggle, Target, H&M, Under the Nile	Hats are especially important if it's chilly in the early days of life, as a lot of heat can escape from baby's unprotected head. If it's summer, get a few sun hats.

Bathing

Item (How Many)	Brands	Tips
Tub (1)	tummy tub, Puj Tub, Stokke Flexi Bath	After the umbilical cord stump falls off, you'll be able to use your tub and fully submerge your baby.
Washcloths or bath mitts (6)	aden & anais, Giggle	Can make sponge baths easier; use one for the face and body and another for the genital area.
Hooded bath towels (2)	Giggle, DwellStudio, Restoration Hardware	Keep the rest of baby wrapped up in the hooded towel while washing parts during sponge baths; the hood keeps baby warm. Get the bigger size—baby will grow fast.
Body wash and body oil (1)	California Baby	Going unscented is probably best. The skin is the largest organ of the body, so going chemical free and organic is a good idea. Body wash should sub in for shampoo at this stage.
Cotton swabs and cotton balls (lots!)	Swisspers Organic	Good for getting into the little chubby folds and creases of the face and body; also great for umbilical care.

Item (How Many)	Brands	Tips
Crystal nail file (1)	Tohar Baby	Much safer than clippers for keeping those tiny nails short. You can file them with ease after a feed or during a nap.
Thermometer (1)	Generation Guard	Take temps in the mouth, on the forehead, or in the armpit.
Snotsucker (1)	Fridababy NoseFrida	Much more gentle than a bulb syringe. Plus you can see if you're getting anything. Remember to buy a pack of filters, too.
Pacifier (4)	Philips Avent Soothies, NUK, Natursutten	Look for cylindrical and single mold. Why single mold? Easy to clean thoroughly. Pacifiers with bells and whistles are tough to clean, and where you can't clean, microbes settle in.
Hairbrush (1)	Fuchs Ambassador Hairbrush	I love this natural wood hairbrush—and not for vanity's sake. Brushing helps stimulate and increase blood flow to the scalp, which is great for little babies. Consider it a scalp massage.
Laundry detergent (one or two bottles to start)	Earth Friendly Products, Seventh Generation	Anything free of fragrance and known irritants.

Diapering

Item (How Many)	Brands	Tips
Disposable diapers (40)	The Honest Company, Parasol, Seventh Generation, Bambo Nature, Eco by Naty	Hold off on buying too many of a single brand in the beginning. It's best to buy a starter amount of two to three brands and see which one fits your baby best. Look for chlorine-free diapers.
Cloth diapers (at least 5 covers and at least 15 inserts or prefolds)	GroVia, Thirsties, bumGenius	The same applies to cloth; do a trial with both before you decide. Also consider a cloth diapering service that might let you try a few different brands at a lower cost.
Diaper pail (1)	Ubbi Steel Diaper Pail	I love this one because there's no special bag required. You can use a standard trash bag and it still locks in odor.
Wipes (5 packs)	The Honest Company, WaterWipes, Naturganics	You can always make your own the first two weeks and transition to store-bought wipes. Look for wipes with limited ingredients.
Reusable cloth wipes (15–30)	Babykicks, Bummis, GroVia	Great if you're cloth diapering or would like to make your own wipes solution and soak the wipes.

Item (How Many)	Brands	Tips
Wipes warmer (1)	Munchkin	Why warm wipes? Warmth feels much better on baby's skin, making diaper changes much less fussy.
Diaper cream (1 tube or bottle)	Motherlove, Boudreaux's Butt Paste, California Baby	When choosing diaper cream, look for a brand that is safe enough to use at every diaper change, if needed, for soothing irritation, keeping skin healthy, and creating a protective barrier against moisture.
Changing pad (1)	Naturepedic	Made from 100% food-grade polyurethane, this nontoxic, water-proof pad is a favorite.

Travel

Item (How Many)	Brands	Tips
Car seat and stroller (1)	UPPAbaby, Britax, Chicco	Look for models that click into your car seat and onto a stroller base, which makes transfers easier with a tiny baby. Consider testing your favorite—if it's too heavy without a baby in it, consider adding 10 to 20 pounds [4.5 to 9 kg] of weight and potentially reconsider your purchase.

>>>

Item (How Many)	Brands	Tips
Soft wrap (1)	Solly Baby Wrap	Great for newborns, as it allows more skin-to-skin interaction; it also can help you get hands-free in those first few weeks. It can be a learning curve to master the wrapping style, but it's no-fuss once you do (look to YouTube for plenty of video tutorials).
Soft structured carrier (1)	Ergobaby	Structured like a backpack, it provides a secure baby-wearing experience. Great as your baby grows and puts on weight and you're needing more support. Look for products that promote the "happy hips" position, which is better for baby's growth.
Diaper bag (1)	Storq, Everlane, Leader Bag Co	Choose a bag that's functional that you enjoy wearing and looking at. You can go that traditional route and get a formal diaper bag, or buy a big hold-all bag and get a few separate bags to put in it.
Portable changing pad (1)	BRICA goPad, Skip Hop	Sleek, utilitarian, easy to clean, and fits in most diaper or non-diaper bags.
Wet bag (1)	Bummis, GroVia	A place to put wet/solid diapers when you're not near a trash can. A roll of dog waste bags are convenient.

Sleep

Item (How Many)	Brands	Tips
Bassinet or cradle cosleeper (1)	SNOO by Happiest Baby, BabyBjörn, Cradle, Snuggle Me Organic	Cosleeping is physiologically compatible with breastfeeding, and if you're not breastfeeding, think night feeds. You'll get more rest sleeping in closer proximity with your baby during those first few weeks. At around three months you can explore shifting to a crib.
Swaddling blankets (4)	aden & anais	The traditional version of the swaddling blanket; you'll use the burrito hold to get your baby comfortably swaddled.
Structured swaddle (4)	aden & anais, Miracle Blanket, Woombie	A simplified version of the traditional swaddle, the structured version makes for easier swaddling, as it usually has panels, Velcro, snaps, or a zipper. Don't commit to one brand before giving it a try with your baby first—they can be awfully particular about these things.
Digital monitor (1)	Nest Cam Indoor security camera	Can be helpful if you would like to look in on your baby when he is sleeping.

Feeding

Item (How Many)	Brands	Tips
Bottles (3)	Dr. Brown's, Comotomo, Playtex Petite VentAire, Minbie, Mixie (for formula)	Choose a slow-flow nipple to avoid over-feeding and pace feed, building in breaks to help with gas.
Drying rack (1)	Boon Grass Countertop Rack, Munchkin Sprout Drying Rack	A separate drying rack for all of your bottle and pumping parts is a good idea; that way things don't get lost or mixed in with your regular family dishes.
Bottle brush (1)	Bürstenhaus Redecker, Oxo Totbottle Brush	Check to see if the company that makes your bottles also makes a brush—in that case the brush is cut to the exact shape of your bottle to make cleaning even easier.
Bottle warmer (1)	Kiinde Kozii	Choose a bottle warmer that best suits the type of feeding you'll be doing. Some warmers are geared toward heating breast milk; others are more appropriate for formula.
Bibs (3)	aden & anais	You'll need a few of these to help stop milk dribbles from getting onto all the cute outfits.
Burp cloths (10)	Giggle	These are great for pretty much everything, not just burping—such as cleaning up spills and standing in as a bib.

Play

Item (How Many)	Brands	Tips
Silk scarves (1 set)	Sarah's Silks	Gently glide it over your baby's face and body as a form of play; it helps develop hand and eye coordination and object permanence.
Soft rattle (2)	Estella, Cheengo	Promotes reaching and auditory development.
Baby gym (1)	Finn + Emma, PlanToys, Skip Hop	Can be used from day one; helps promote physical and cognitive development.
Sheepskin blanket (1)	ecowool	Make sure that it's pesticide-free; skins make a cozy play mat that helps regulate your baby's temperature. Great for underneath their back while playing in the gym.
Board books (2)	*Goodnight Moon, Where Is Baby's Belly Button?*	Use as part of pre-nap or pre-bedtime routines. Try books that have a sing-songy rhythm, a phrase that's repeated over and over, or ones that aren't too visually overwhelming.

Breastfeeding

Item (How Many)	Brands	Tips
Double expression personal breast pump (1)	Medela Pump In Style, Spectra S2	Medela is the best-known brand in the U.S., but Spectra is an excellent alternative at lower cost
Double expression hospital cradle pump (1)	Medela Symphony, Spectra Baby S1	Rent or purchase this type if you're having any issues breastfeeding immediately after birth; these pumps are strong enough to help stimulate your milk supply.
Single expression hand pump (1)	Medela	Great for night pumping sessions; it allows for quick, easy, and quiet pumping and can live easily on your bedside table. With this you can pump only one breast at a time. Can be helpful during engorgement.
Pumping bags (25)	Kiinde Twist Pouches, Lansinoh Bags, Freemie Collection Cups	Twist Pouches are leak-proof, so they eliminate messy and risky transfer of milk, and I love that they have a lid. BPA-free, phtalate-free, and PVC-free. Lansinoh Bags are great because they lie flat; store, freeze, thaw, and pour well; are easy to transport; and hardly ever leak, due to their double zipper seal. Presterilized and BPA-free.

Item (How Many)	Brands	Tips
Breast milk storage organizer (1)	Kiinde	The Kiinde Keeper helps with storing breast milk in an organized, protected, and safe way. Breast milk storage bags can lie flat in one of the twelve compartments, which makes freezing, thawing, and warming easier. It takes up minimal space in the freezer or refrigerator, and protects bags from puncture damage or sticking together while freezing. Bags can also be easily organized by date. It's meant to work with Kiinde Twist Pouches, but can work with most breast milk storage bags.
Breast shields (2 sets of 2)	Buy according to the pump you buy or try Freemies	Most pumps come with their standard size breast shield, and few other size options. Comfortable shields = happy pumping.
Nursing bra (4)	Cosabella, Bravado, Cake, Yummie by Heather Thomson	Purchase about a month before your due date; by then you'll be at your fullest breast size before having your baby, and your rib cage will have reached its maximum expansion.

>>>

Item (How Many)	Brands	Tips
Sleep bra (1)	Storq, Cake	Provides less support than a typical nursing bra, but makes for easy night feeds and allows you to use nursing pads to contain night leakage.
Hands-free pumping bra (1)	Simple Wishes	This bra allows you to pump hands free, so you can get hands on and incorporate breast massage to help maximize your yield.
Nursing pads (1 package)	Disposable: Lansinoh Reusable: Bamboobies	You'll need these to help catch any leakage during the day or as you sleep.
Leak-proof nursing pads (1 set)	LilyPadz	If you leak a lot, these are a great option. Made of silicone, they help stop leaks before they happen.
Milkies Milk-Saver (1 set)	Milkies	Helps collect and store up to 10 additional ounces of breast milk a day, and it reduces the need for disposable nursing pads. While your baby is nursing on one breast, place this on the other breast to collect leaks.
Breastfeeding pillow (1 set)	Ergobaby	Look for a nursing pillow that is fairly firm; that way your baby won't sink into the pillow.

Item (How Many)	Brands	Tips
Nipple cream (1)	Motherlove	Look for a vegan, non-lanolin-based nipple cream with food-based ingredients—most nipple creams don't have to be removed in between feeds.
Hydrogels (1)	Ameda	Helps soothe sore nipples by reducing contact with the clothing or bra fabric. Pop them in the fridge to cool them before and in between uses.
Hot and cold compresses (1 set)	Earth Mama Angel Baby Booby Tubes	Warm, moist heat before nursing and a cold compress after or in between feeds can be a big help during engorgement. A warm compress while pumping can help increase your yield. These natural, safe, gel-free breast packs are made with a 100-percent organic cotton shell and filled with flax seeds.
Nipple repair (1 set)	Silverette	Small nursing cups made out of 925 silver help protect the nipples while breastfeeding. Silver is a natural anti-microbial and anti-inflammatory element; it heals cuts, wounds, cracks, and soreness, and prevents infections.

>>>

Item (How Many)	Brands	Tips
Nipple everter/ protection (1 set)	TheraShells by Medela	You can place these on your nipples to help protect them in between feeds if they feel painful or raw; they also allow air to flow around the nipple. They can also help your nipples to evert if they are flat or inverted.

Postpartum Goods

Item (How Many)	Brands	Tips
Sitz bath bowl (1)	Yungatart Seatz Bath	A sitz bath bowl is a warm, shallow bath that cleanses the perineum. Sitting in a sitz bath and adding herbs and water or another liquid herbal solution can provide much relief after labor. Make sure to wash the bath thoroughly after each use. There is a DIY herbal sitz bath recipe to use with your bowl on page 296.
Witch hazel pads (1)	Thayers Natural Remedies	Provides instant relief when placed on swollen tissues. Great for hemorrhoids.

Item (How Many)	Brands	Tips
Peri bottle (1)	Fridababy's Fridet MomWasher	Helps reduce stinging in the perineum when you urinate, caused by the uric acid in urine as it runs over raw skin. Remember to squeeze the solution on while you urinate. Unlike most peri bottles, this one is designed to be held upside down.
Donut cushion (1)	Kieba	Helps take pressure off the perineum so sitting is more comfortable.
Disposable underwear (1 package)	Depends Silhouette	These are soft and comfortable, don't pull at anything, and hold everything in, which can be very helpful overnight for lochia and incontinence.
Maxi pads (1 pack)	Natracare	If you'd prefer to forgo the Depends route, I like these organic maxi pads.
Leak-proof underwear (3 or 4)	Thinx, Icon Undies	A more lightweight option for the end of your lochia period.
High-waisted underwear/shapewear (2–4)	Total Comfort (TC) Fine Intimates, Yummie by Heather Thomson	Great for helping you feel more collected and comfortable while your swelling improves.

Belly Care

Item (How Many)	Brands	Tips
Belly band (1)	McDavid Waist Trimmer Belly Bandit Body Formulate Fit (BFF)	Using a belly band or shaping high-waisted underwear can help make you feel more collected, supporting your back and making it easier to hold your baby and do other tasks. I like the McDavid Waist Trimmer; it's neoprene inside, which allows you to sweat—a boon in the first few days. The Belly Bandit is another option made from a breathable modal fabric.
Belly balm or oil (1)	Zoe Organics, organic coconut oil	Keep up with gentle massage and lubrication of the belly. There is a DIY body oil recipe on page 311.

Cesarean Birth Recovery

Item (How Many)	Brand	Tips
Recovery underwear (1)	C-Panty	Compression underwear with a medical-grade silicone panel over the incision area to speed healing and reduce swelling; also supports tissue that has been weakened by surgery. Get consent from your care provider before using the C-Panty.

Item	Brand	Tips
Incision healing salve (1)	Earth Mother Angel Baby	Use in the evening to help with scar healing. Get consent from your care provider before using any creams or oils near or on the incision area or to recommend a prescription cream.

ASSEMBLING YOUR PREFERENCES

There's so much to consider when it comes to your birth team, environment, and preferred procedures. What follows is a checklist of various birth procedures and an example of the preferences grid you should provide for your caregiver(s).

This checklist is designed to help you organize your thoughts about your birth experiences and formulate your preferences. Use the options here to work through and consider what elements of your pending birthing experience are important to you—and what things you're open to changing. Remember: Realistic preferences embrace flexibility.

Starting or Speeding Labor

Natural Induction Methods

- ○ Walking
- ○ Acupressure
- ○ Nipple stimulation
- ○ Chiropractic adjustment
- ○ Castor oil
- ○ Sex

Medical Induction Methods

- ○ Prostaglandin medications
- ○ Membrane sweep
- ○ AROM (artificial rupture of membranes)
- ○ Pitocin
- ○ Foley bulb

Monitoring During Labor

- ○ Intermittent
- ○ Continuous

>>>

Hydration and Nourishment

○ IV fluids   ○ Saline lock   ○ No IV

Desired foods:

○ ....   ○ ....   ○ ....

○ ....   ○ ....   ○ ....

○ ....   ○ ....   ○ ....

Desired drinks:

○ ....   ○ ....   ○ ....

○ ....   ○ ....   ○ ....

○ ....   ○ ....   ○ ....

Pain Relief

Relaxation Techniques

○ Walking   ○ Visualization   ○ Vocalization

○ Breathing   ○ Massage   ○ Hydrotherapy

Narcotics

○ Only if requested   ○ Offer as soon as possible   ○ Do not offer

Epidural

○ Offer as soon as possible   ○ Do not offer

Environment

○ Location: ....   ○ Temperature: ....   ○ Aromatherapy/ essential oils: ....

○ Lighting: ....   ○ Music: ....   ○ Clothing: ....

Positions

Upright

- ⭘ Walking
- ⭘ Lunging
- ⭘ Leaning on wall/ person
- ⭘ Sitting on ball
- ⭘ Squatting with support

Hands and Knees

- ⭘ With ball
- ⭘ On bed
- ⭘ Pelvic rocking

Reclining

- ⭘ Active rest

Pushing Possibilities

Positions

- ⭘ Squatting
- ⭘ Standing
- ⭘ Hands and knees
- ⭘ Reclining

Method

- ⭘ Spontaneous
- ⭘ Directed

Perineal Care

- ⭘ Support
- ⭘ Massage
- ⭘ Compresses
- ⭘ Positioning
- ⭘ Episiotomy

Support

- ⭘ Partner
- ⭘ Doula
- ⭘ Family member(s): _____

_____

_____

_____

Newborn Procedures

- ○ Eye ointment
- ○ Vitamin K
- ○ Hepatitis B
- ○ PKU
- ○ Cord blood banking
- ○ Delayed cord clamping
- ○ Circumcision

Placenta

- ○ Using
- ○ Not using

Cesarean Birth

Anesthesia

- ○ Epidural
- ○ Spinal block
- ○ General anesthesia

Process

- ○ Describe events
- ○ Video/photos
- ○ Skin to skin immediately

Birth Preferences Grid

I know labor and delivery units—and I know what doctors and nurses find useful. It's a single sheet of paper that they can glance at and refer to periodically—not your life story. Once you've determined your birth preferences, create a document similar to the following example. (It is only an example of someone else's completed grid, not recommendations for how to fill out your own grid!) Print two copies and pack them in your hospital bag. Even if you're birthing at home or a birth center, have your preferences ready for the hospital, in case you need to transfer. Discuss your preferences with your doctor or midwife to make sure they're apprised of your wants long before you go into labor.

Your Name and Your Partner's Name

Your Birth Team: *OB/GYN, Midwife, Doula, Pediatrician*

Goal: Healthy Mother and Healthy Baby

Starting Labor

Nonmedical Induction Methods:
Walking, acupuncture, acupressure, sex, chiropractic adjustment

Medical Induction:
We are open to: *membranes sweep, Cervidil, Cytotec, Foley bulb, breaking my water, Pitocin*

Low-risk method preferred. Please explain all options before proceeding.

During Labor

Monitoring:
Intermittent; Doppler, if available

No IV or IV fluids, unless medically necessary

Food and Drink:
Access to liquids/ice according to thirst

Permission to eat brought food, according to labor

Environment
Low lights and aromatherapy

Pain Management

Relaxation Techniques:
Breathwork, low lights

Movement:
Unmedicated: I would like to move freely and use a birth ball, peanut ball, massage, and aromatherapy.

Medicated: I am open to an epidural, but please only offer it when I request it.

Pushing and Delivery

Spontaneous, with varied positions

Perineal Care
Guided pushing and positioning; counterpressure; massage with mineral oil

No episiotomy unless medically necessary—to be decided only by my doctor, not by a resident

Cesarean Birth

Partner present in OR

Spinal block preferred over general anesthesia

Mom and baby together for recovery/skin to skin immediately following delivery

If mother is unable, please have partner do skin to skin

Newborn Care

Delay cord-clamping and cutting

Quick transfer to mother for skin to skin and for as long as possible (45 minutes to 1 hour)

Donate cord blood

Breastfeeding

Allow/assist mother to breastfeed within 2 hours of delivery

No pacifier/bottle or formula. If mother is asleep for feeding, please wake her up.

Placenta

Please save for encapsulation

LABOR PREP GUIDE

One Month Before Due Date

Evening Primrose Oil

Preliminary research suggests that this may be helpful in softening the cervix prior to labor. The active ingredient is linoleic acid, which helps make prostaglandins (the chemical made by your body when it's ready for labor). As of yet there are no identified side effects.

Try: Take 1000 mg (1 gram) once daily; increase to three times daily two weeks before your due date. Metagenics is a great brand.

Red Raspberry Leaf

A uterine tonic, this tea prepares the uterus to contract effectively, yet it is not associated with causing preterm labor. It has been associated with decreased complications for both mother and baby.

Try: The Nettle Raspberry Infusion on page 98 in a daily dose.

Acupuncture

Treatments can be centered around decreasing anxiety, guiding your baby into an optimal position, ripening the cervix, and relaxing the pelvic muscles. Check with your acupuncturist beforehand to see if she's familiar with labor prep techniques—and make sure to ask how many women she's helped start labor!

Try: Weekly prebirth treatments starting around weeks 35 to 37.

Over 40 Weeks?

Chiropractic Adjustment

Consider seeing a licensed chiropractor; they can use a method called the Webster technique, which can help make sure that your sacrum and supporting muscles, ligaments, and joints are free of restriction and imbalance, which can help your labor begin. This adjustment consists of a physical sacral rotation and then a gentle trigger point pressure of opposite sides of the round ligament, which helps support your uterus along with the broad ligament.

Acupuncture

Acupuncture can be very effective for starting labor if you're past your due date. Daily treatments will probably be recommended. If it's going to work, you could have labor signs after one treatment, but more commonly after two or three treatments.

Clary Sage Bath

Clary sage is a powerful uterine stimulant, so it should not be used before your due date, as it can help start contractions. Add at least ten to fifteen drops to a warm bath. Breathe deeply and try to relax (and not think about your due date).

Try: As often as you like within that week. Continue with the techniques already listed.

Sex

Semen contains prostaglandins, which, when they contact the cervix, can help it soften. Plus, orgasms release oxytocin, which can help promote contractions. If your water hasn't broken and you still feel amorous, go for it!

CELEBRATING YOUR PREGNANCY, YOUR BIRTH, AND YOUR BABY

To shower or not to shower? It can be somewhat complicated. Maybe you're close with your family, who would be most comfortable throwing you a traditional baby shower, but you and your partner would prefer a more inclusive, gender-neutral celebration sans the silly games. Or maybe you'd love something for just your girlfriends, but the usual party ideas feel pretty stale and not you at all. No worries—here are a handful of ideas to make a shower, blessingway, or gender-inclusive new-baby celebration completely your own.

The traditional shower You may feel like marching to the beat of your own drum, but one of the biggest things you'll learn about becoming a new mother is the power of family. If yours wants to throw you a baby shower—complete with pink or blue balloons, ribbons, diaper games, and all manner of things you genuinely dislike—I say go for it. It may not be your aesthetic, but hey, they are your people. You may not love the trappings, but I can almost guarantee that you'll feel the love. Depending on your relationships, that could be better than the perfectly Instagrammable party.

The nontraditional shower As mothers, we ask more of our partners than in previous generations—and now they want in on the baby celebrations! In truth, if you're hoping for a solid coparenting relationship, a great way to start is a coparented baby shower. The paradigm for this type of party is yet to be set, so do whatever feels right for you as a couple: a backyard barbecue, a sit-down dinner, passed appetizers at a restaurant you love, an outdoor screening of *Parenthood*, or hey, a traditional shower, but inclusive of all genders—whatever feels right is right.

The blessingway A popular alternative to the traditional baby shower, a blessingway (inspired by a Navajo tradition) is a time for a mother-to-be to gather with those who are close to her, traditionally all women (although anyone who is sincerely close to the woman should be welcomed). These ceremonies are less involved with celebrating the new baby and more focused on supporting the mother in her journey through pregnancy and wishing her well for the birth. Events include supportive exercises, like pampering the new mother. I'm particularly fond of creating a birth necklace. Each participant brings a bead and a blessing for the new mother (friends and family who live far away often send theirs ahead of time). At the blessingway, each guest says their blessing and gifts the bead to the mother-to-be. After the blessingway, the new mother creates the necklace, or a friend or family member does it for her, and she wears this necklace as a reminder of the strength and power of her community—and their confidence in her.

Building Your Registry and Extra Help

Hopefully The Goods list has given you a fair amount of help in starting your registry. Even so, you may still want a few more resources. Here are a few tried-and-true options for building your registry.

BabyList This site is an easy and seamless way to create an online registry from multiple websites. (babylist.com)

Giggle A great resource for all manner of new baby essentials. Plus, they even have a registry app to make sure you check off everything on the list!

BabyGearLab My favorite site for researching baby products and gear (especially strollers, bottles, and car seats). Reviewers purchase items at retail (no gifts or samples from manufacturers) and give honest, thorough write-ups on their thoughts. It's a great place to look if you're stuck between a few options. (babygearlab.com)

Labor support If you're interested in working with a doula or your insurance doesn't cover all of the birthing options you'd prefer (say, birthing at home), consider adding a monetary gift option to your registry. It's fairly easy to set up on most registry sites these days (BabyList makes it quite easy) and is a great way to get some extra mother support.

Giving back Prepping for a new baby can be expensive, and the majority of new mothers could use the help. However, if you're financially comfortable to do so, a wonderful thing to do is to redirect gift-givers to a local charity in support of mothers and babies in need. They can purchase items and donate to places like BabyToBaby or make cash donations in the name of your new baby, which is a great way to encourage a lifetime of stewardship.

For more tips on ways you can direct your community to help, flip back to Chapter Eleven (page 284) and read the sections on Guests and Family, and Getting Help.

FEELING STRESSED? LET'S ASSESS.

In Chapter Eleven, we explored the different mood disorders that can occur postpartum. Doctors and therapists alike are starting to see that postpartum anxiety and postpartum depression are not totally distinct; in fact, anxiety could perpetuate depression. Below is a list of scenarios taken from a postpartum assessment tool published in 2011 in the *Journal of Women's Health* that incorporates both feelings of anxiety and depression. If you are reading this postpartum and notice that you've been feeling more stressed or upset than usual, find a moment when your baby is sleeping to scan it. If more than one of the following scenarios apply to you, talk to your care provider, your partner, or a friend sooner rather than later. Don't let shame, finances, uncertainty, or denial get in the way of you getting the support you might need.

- I feel sad and hopeless.

- I am crying more than usual.

- I cannot make decisions or concentrate.

- I feel overwhelmed.

- I have recurring thoughts about my baby getting sick or having some kind of problem.

- I check on my baby multiple times throughout the night.

- I have thoughts about my baby that scare me.

- I think about taking my own life.

- I'm afraid I will never feel better.

Acknowledgments

To my husband and best friend, Jordy, for encouraging me as the book came to fruition. I love you and can't wait for all that's to come for us and our future family. You saw this before I did.

To Zinzi Edmundson, for being my left brain on this book and helping me anchor my never-ending stream of thoughts. Your patience and acceptance of my voice, notes, and basically just "getting it" made the writing process a labor of love. I'm lucky to call you a dear friend. PS: Your approach to motherhood is 100 percent #goals. Can't tell you how proud of you I am. I'm grateful that James brought us together.

To Dr. Suzanne Gilberg-Lenz, for your friendship and holistic wisdom.

To my father, for being the truest example of dedication, intelligence, and hard work; I wouldn't be here without your love and support.

To my mother, thank you for birthing me into this world.

To my agent, Kari Stuart, thank you for being a sounding board and cheerleader on this long road. I have a feeling that there is more in store. You helped make this easier. No doubt.

To the Chronicle team, thank you for shepherding me through this process and believing that I was the right person to write this book. I'm forever grateful.

Trademarks

Aden & Anais is a registered trademark of Aden & Anais, Inc. Ameda is a registered trademark of Ameda, Inc. Baby To Baby is a registered trademark of Baby To Baby. BabyBjörn is a registered trademark of BabyBjörn AB. BabyGearLab is a registered trademark of BabyGearLab LLC. BabyKicks is a registered trademark of ITC Services LLC DBA BabyKicks LLC. Babylist is a registered trademark of Babylist. Bach's Flower Remedies: White Chestnut, Red Chestnut, Rescue Remedy, are registered trademarks of Nelson & Co Ltd. Bambo Nature is a registered trademark of Bambo Nature by Abena. Bamboobies is a registered trademark of Soft Style Inc. Belly Bandit Upsie Belly is a registered trademark of Belly Bandit. Blanqi is a registered trademark of Blanqi LLC. Boudreaux's Butt Paste is a registered trademark of CB Fleet. Bravado is a registered trademark of Medela Holding AG Corp. Switzerland. BRICA is a registered trademark of Munchkin. Britax is a registered trademark of Britax. Bugaboo is a registered trademark of Bugaboo International B.V. bumGenius is a registered trademark of Cotton Babies, Inc. Bummis is a registered trademark of Bummis. Bürstenhaus Redecker is a registered trademark of Burstenhaus Redecker. C-Panty is a registered trademark of UpSpring. Cake Maternity is a registered trademark of Cake Maternity. California Baby is a registered trademark of Ralph, Paco & Roberto, Inc. Carter's is a registered trademark of Carter's, Inc. Cervidil is a registered trademark of Ferring B.V. Cheengo is a registered trademark of Cheengo. Comotomo is a registered trademark of Cosabella. CrossFit is a registered trademark of CrossFit, Inc. Cytotec is a registered trademark of Pfizer Inc. Demerol is a registered trademark of sanofi-aventis U.S. LLC. Depends is a registered trademark of Kimberly-Clark Worldwide, Inc. DockATot is a registered trademark of Enfant Terrible Design AB LLC. Dr. Brown's is a registered trademark of Handi-Craft Company. Dwellstudio is a registered trademark of dwellstudio. Earth Friendly Products is a registered trademark of Venus Laboratories, Inc. Earth Mama Angel Baby Booby Tubes is a registered trademark of Earth Mama. Eco by Naty is a registered trademark of Naty AB. ecowool is a registered trademark of ecowool. Environmental Working Group and Skin Deep Database are registered trademarks of EWG. Epsoak is a registered trademark of San Francisco Salt Co. Ergobaby is a registered trademark of Ergobaby. Estella is a registered trademark of Estella. Etsy is a registered trademark of Etsy Co. Everlane is a registered trademark of Everlane, Inc. Ezekiel is a registered trademark of Food For Life. Facebook is a registered trademark of Facebook, Inc. Finn + Emma is a registered trademark of Finn + Emma. Flexi bath is a registered trademark of Stokke AS. Floracopeia is a registered trademark of Floracopeia. Floradix is a registered trademark of Nature's Synergy Pty Ltd. Freemie is a registered trademark of Dao Health Co. Fridababy, NosaFrida, and Fridet MomWasher are registered trademarks of Fridababy LLC. Fuchs Ambassador Hairbrush is a registered trademark of FUCHS GmbH Co. Generation Guard is a registered trademark of Generation Guard Pty Ltd. Giggle is a registered trademark of giggle. Great Lakes Collagen Powder is a registered trademark of Great Lakes Gelatin Company. GroVia is a registered trademark of The Natural Baby Company, LLC. Google is a registered trademark of Google Inc. H&M is a registered trademark of Hennes & Mauritz AB Co. Hatch is a registered trademark of Hatch Collection. The Honest Company is a registered trademark of The Honest Company. Icon Undies and Thinx are registered trademarks of THINX Inc. Instagram is a registered trademark of Instagram LLC. KellyMom Online is a registered trademark of KellyMom.com. Kieba is a registered trademark of Pharm Logistics, Inc. Kiinde Kozii is a registered trademark of Kiinde, Inc. La Leche League is a registered trademark of La Leche League International. Lansinoh is a registered trademark of Lansinoh Laboratories, Inc. Leader Bag Co is a registered trademark of Leader Bag Co., LLC. Life-flo is a registered trademark of NutraMarks, Inc. LilyPadz is a registered trademark of Me & My Kidz, LLC. McDavid is a registered trademark of McDavid. Meal Train is a registered trademark of Meal Train LLC. Medela Pump in Style is a registered trademark of Medela, Inc. MegaFood is a registered trademark of FoodState, Inc. Metagenics: Wellness Essentials Pregnancy is a registered trademark of Metagenics, Inc. Milkies is a registered trademark of Fairhaven Health, LLC. Minbie is a registered trademark of Minbie US. Miracle Blanket is a registered trademark of Miracle Industries, LLC. Mixie is a registered trademark of Mixie. Motherlove is a registered trademark of Motherlove Herbal Company. Mountain Rose Herbs is a registered trademark of Mountain Rose Herbs. Munchkin is a registered trademark of Munchkin Inc. Natracare is a registered trademark of Bodywise (UK) Limited. Natural Calm and Natural Vitality are registered trademarks of Natural Vitality. Naturepedic is a registered trademark of BJ2, LLC. NatureWise Women's Care is a registered trademark of NatureWise. Naturganics is a registered trademark of Brashears, David R. Naturganic Distrobutors Individual. Natursutten is a registered trademark of EcoBaby ApS LLC. Nest is a registered trademark of Nest Labs. New Chapter is a registered trademark of P&G. NUK is a registered trademark of NUK USA LLC. Oxo is a registered trademark of Helen of Troy Limited. Parasol is a registered trademark of Parasol Co. Patagonia is a registered trademark of Patagonia, Inc. Periscope is a registered trademark of Twitter, Inc. Philips Advent Soothie is a registered trademark of Koninklijke Philips N.V. Pitocin is a registered trademark of JP Pharmaceuticals. PJ's Bliss is a registered trademark of Limerick Inc. PlanToys is a registered trademark of PlanToys. Playtex is a registered trademark of Playtex Marketing Corporation. Polarn O. Pyret is a registered trademark of Polarn O. Pyret. Preggers is a registered trademark of Therafirm.com. Preparation H is a registered trademark of Pfizer Consumer Healthcare. Primary is a registered trademark of Primary Kids, Inc. Puj Tub is a registered trademark of Puj. Rainbow Light Advanced Enzyme Optima is a registered trademark of Rainbow Light. Restoration Hardware is a registered trademark of Restoration Hardware, Inc. Ryvita is a registered trademark of The Ryvita Company Limited. Sarah's Silks is a registered trademark of Sarah's Silks. Seventh Generation is a registered trademark of Seventh Generation, Inc. Silverette is a registered trademark of Tecnologia Ospedaliera S.r.l. LLC. Simple Wishes is a registered trademark of Simple Wishes, LLC. Skip Hop is a registered trademark of Skip Hop. Snapchat is a registered trademark of Snapchat, Inc. SNOO by Happiest Baby is a registered trademark of Happiest Baby Inc. Snow Lotus Aromatherapy is a registered trademark of Snow Lotus Aromatherapy. Solly Baby is a registered trademark of Solly Baby, Inc. Source Naturals is a registered trademark of Source Naturals, Inc. Storq is a registered trademark of Storq. Swisspers Organic is a registered trademark of U.S. Cotton, LLC. Target is a registered trademark of Target Brand Inc. Thayers Natural Remedies is a registered trademark of Thayers Natural Remedies. TheraShells is a registered trademark of Medela, Inc. Thirsties is a registered trademark of Thirsties, Inc. Tohar Baby is a registered trademark of Tohar Baby. Total Comfort Fine Intimates is a registered trademark of Classic Shapewear. Tummy tub is a registered trademark of tummy tub. Ubbi is a registered trademark of ubbiworld. Under the Nile is a registered trademark of Under the Nile. UPPAbaby is a registered trademark of UPPAbaby. Vitals is a registered trademark of Vitals. WaterWipes is a registered trademark of Irish Breeze Limited. Whole Foods is a registered trademark of Whole Foods Market IP. L.P. WishGarden is a registered trademark of WishGarden Herbal Remedies. Woombie is a registered trademark of KB Designs LLC. Yelp is a registered trademark of Yelp Inc. YouTube is a registered trademark of Google Inc. Yummie by Heather Thomson is a registered trademark of Yummie Life. Yungatart Seatz Bath is a registered trademark of Yungatart. Zara is a registered trademark of Inditex. Zoe Organics is a registered trademark of Zoe Organics.

Index